Challenges in the Treatment of Congenital Cardiac Anomalies

Challenges in the Treatment of Congenital Cardiac Anomalies

Edited by

Masato Takahashi, M.D.

Associate Professor of Pediatrics
University of Southern California School of Medicine
Director, Cardiac Catheterization Laboratory
Childrens Hospital of Los Angeles
Los Angeles, California

Winfield J. Wells, M.D.

Associate Clinical Professor of Surgery
University of Southern California School of Medicine
Los Angeles, California

George G. Lindesmith, M.D.

Clinical Professor of Surgery
University of Southern California School of Medicine
Head, Division of Thoracic and Cardiovascular Surgery
Childrens Hospital of Los Angeles
Los Angeles, California

Library of Congress Cataloging-in-Publication Data

Challenges in the treatment of congenital cardiac
  anomalies.

  Includes bibliographies and index.
  1. Heart—Abnormalities—Treatment.   2. Pediatric
cardiology.   I. Takahashi, Masato, 1933–
II. Lindesmith, George G. (George Gerald), 1928–
III. Wells, Winfield J. [DNLM: 1. Heart Defects,
Congenital—therapy. WS 290 C437]
RJ421.C47   1986   618.92'12043   86-45769
ISBN 0-87993-220-1

Published by
Futura Publishing Company, Inc.
P.O. Box 330, 295 Main Street
Mount Kisco, New York 10549

L.C. No.: 86-45769
ISBN No.: 0-87993-220-1

Contributors

Bailey, Leonard L., MD., Chief, Pediatric Cardiac Surgery, Assistant Professor of Surgery and Pediatrics, Loma Linda University School of Medicine, Loma Linda, California.

Baño-Rodrigo, Antonio, M.D., Research Fellow, Cardiac Pathology, The Children's Hospital, Boston, Massachusetts.

Bing, Richard J., M.D., Professor of Medicine (Emeritus), University of Southern California School of Medicine, Los Angeles, California; Director Experimental Cardiology and Scientific Development, Huntington Medical Research Institutes; Visiting Associate in Chemistry, California Institute of Technology, Pasadena, California.

Danielson, Gordon K., M.D., Consultant, Division of Thoracic and Cardiovascular Surgery, Professor of Surgery, Mayo Medical School, Rochester, Minnesota.

Fyler, Donald C., M.D., Associate Professor of Pediatrics, Harvard Medical School; Associate Chief, Cardiology, Children's Hospital Medical Center, Boston, Massachusetts.

Gersony, Welton, M.D., Profesor of Pediatrics and Director, Division of Pediatric Cardiology, Columbia—Presbyterian Medical Center, New York, New York.

Hohn, Arno R., M.D., Professor of Pediatrics, University of Southern California School of Medicine; Head, Division of Cardiology, Childrens Hospital, Los Angeles, California.

Lababidi, Zuhdi, M.D., Professor and Director, Pediatric Cardiology,

University of Missouri Hospital and Clinics, Department of Child Health, Columbia, Missouri.

Lewis, Alan B., M.D., Associate Professor of Pediatrics, University of Southern California School of Medicine; Director of Cardiology Training and Research, Childrens Hospital, Los Angeles, California.

Lock, James E., M.D., Associate Professor of Pediatrics, Pediatric Cardiology, Department of Cardiology, Children's Hospital Medical Center, Boston, Massachusetts.

Matsuoka, Rumiko, M.D., Research Fellow, Children's Hospital Medical Center, Department of Cardiac Pathology, Boston, Massachusetts.

Pacifico, Albert D., M.D., Professor of Surgery, University of Alabama Department of Surgery, Birmingham, Alabama.

Schuetz, Thomas J., Medical Student, Research Student, Cardiac Pathology, Harvard Medical School, Boston, Massachusetts.

Smolinsky, Aram, M.D., Instructor in Surgery, Harvard Medical School, Boston, Massachusetts.

Stanton, Robert E., M.D., Associate Professor of Pediatrics, University of Southern California School of Medicine; Associate Head, Division of Cardiology, Coordinator Undergraduate Student Education, Childrens Hospital, Los Angeles, California

Turley, Kevin, M.D., Associate Professor, Department of Surgery, University of California, San Francisco, California.

Van Praagh, Richard, M.D., Professor of Pathology, Research Associate in Cardiology, Children's Hospital, Harvard Medical School, Boston, Massachusetts.

Van Praagh, Stella, M.D., Assistant Professor in Pathology, Associate in Cardiology, Children's Hospital Medical Center, Harvard Medical School, Boston, Massachusetts.

Preface

This book is intended for pediatric cardiologists, cardiac surgeons, and other physicians involved in the treatment of congenital heart disease. It is neither an exhaustive textbook nor a strict monograph on one subject. Rather, this volume is meant to fill a certain void. As we go about the daily business of taking care of children with heart diseases, we feel the need, from time to time, to review certain subject matters in sufficient depth and in a systematic fashion so as to bolster our working knowledge of the subject and to put into a proper perspective knowledge we have accumulated through random reading of journals and listening to papers at medical meetings. We have chosen four areas of current interest, the left heart obstructive lesions, transposition of the great arteries, truncus arteriosus, and balloon angioplasty. With the exception of balloon angioplasty, each area was discussed by a pathologist, cardiologist, and a number of surgeons, in sequence, in order to move our thought process from morphology to physiology to medical and surgical management. Assessment of outcome and alternatives in treatment are fully addressed.

The leading chapter "Congenital Heart Disease: Beginnings" by Dr. Richard Bing has been included to remind us of the efforts of our pioneers. In this connection, we are particularly saddened to learn of the recent death of Dr. Helen Taussig. Pediatric cardiology began with Dr. Taussig. She has influenced all of us immeasurably through the formative years of our discipline.

This volume is the fourth in the series of similar books to come out of the cardiovascular service at Children's Hospital of Los Angeles since 1979. Although both the impetus and material for publication come from our conferences held every other year in Los Angeles, we have taken great pains to make our books pertinent and readable to all practitioners of the art. (For those readers who wish to examine previous publications in this series references follow.)

vii

The editors wish to thank Mrs. Margaret Stevenson of the Heart and Lung Surgery Foundation of Los Angeles for the preparation of manuscripts and to Mr. Steven Korn and Mrs. Helen Powers of Futura Publishing Company for their valuable advice.

Masato Takahashi, M.D.
Winfield J. Wells, M.D.
George G. Lindesmith, M.D.

References

Tucker BL, Lindesmith GG (eds): *First Clinical Conference on Congenital Heart Disease*. New York, Grune & Stratton, 1979.

Tucker BL, Lindesmith GG, Takahashi, M (eds): *Second Clinical Conference on Congenital Heart Disease*. New York, Grune & Stratton, 1982.

Tucker BL, Lindesmith GG, Takahashi, M (eds): *Obstructive Lesions of the Right Heart. Third Clinical Conference on Congenital Heart Disease*. Baltimore, University Park Press, 1983.

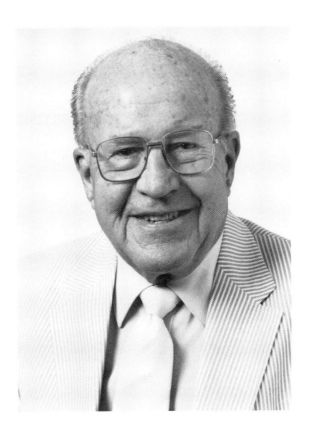

*This volume is dedicated to Bert Wiley Meyer,
an active cardiovascular surgeon who pioneered
cardiac surgery at the Childrens Hospital of Los
Angeles in the early 1950s. His experience has
spanned the prepump era up to and including the
current techniques, and his contributions to the
cardiac surgical program at the Childrens Hospital
have been instrumental to its success. He has been
directly involved in training most of us who are
active in the cardiac surgical program, and his
continued active participation is an asset of
immeasurable value to all of us involved in the
treatment of congenital heart disease at the
Childrens Hospital.*

Contents

Section III.   Transposition of the Great Arteries

Section I

Historical Perspectives

The development of the heart . . . is very complex . . . from what was once just atoms dispersed in space, this beautiful heart develops automatically, and is perfectly normal at birth 99.4% of the time.

Dwight C. McGoon, M.D.
Ecstasy

CHAPTER 1

Congenital Heart Disease: Beginnings

Richard J. Bing, M.D.

History, whether that of nations, arts, science, or medicine, is formed by the famous and the unsung. Often the difference between fame and oblivion for an individual depends on the circumstances rather than on qualifications. This applies to congenital heart disease which, within the recent past, owes much to the well-known and famous. However, the contributions, of the early anatomists, who were the first to contribute were almost forgotten. The knowledge of congenital heart disease is founded on anatomy. It was necessary to understand fully the normal anatomy of the heart before pathological anatomy could be recognized and appreciated. To this day pathological anatomical exploration of the heart is in progress. The second phase of our knowledge of congenital heart disease has been contingent upon the advent of surgical therapy. It is characterized by studies of changes in circulation and physiological adaptation to the malformation. The third phase, which overlaps the others, emphasizes improved diagnosis and surgical treatment. It is entirely based on technological advances.

The first contribution to our knowledge of congenital heart disease was the anatomical nature of the malformation; this could take place only after the normal anatomy and function had been understood. With Vesalius, Harvey, and Vieussens the fundamental anatomical concepts had been formulated.

One of the rediscovered, unsung heroes of this early phase is Niels Stensen, the real discoverer of the malformation that now bears Fallot's name. As a fellow working in Copenhagen, Denmark, in the early 1930s, my colleague, E. Warburg, referred to the "tetralogy of Stensen" rather than that of Fallot. Who was Niels Stensen? He is best remembered because of his discovery of the parotid duct, now known as Stensen's duct. His life reflects the turbulence of the seventeenth

3

century with its religious and political strife in which the vestiges of the late Renaissance still lingered and the Baroque demanded to be born. At the University of Copenhagen, among the pictures of the early anatomists there hangs a portrait of a Catholic bishop, Niels Stensen; however, Stensen is not buried in Denmark, but in the tombs of the Medici in the Basilica of St. Lawrence in Florence, Italy. How did it happen that a Danish anatomist became a Catholic bishop and was buried with the Medicis in Florence?

Stensen was born in Copenhagen in 1638. He studied at the University of Copenhagen under the famous anatomist, Bartholin. He then moved to Leyden, where he worked with Silvius. In Holland he discovered the parotid duct, which bears his name. Controversies as to the priority of this discovery soon arose, and Stensen left for home in 1664. It is here that he became preoccupied with the heart. A remarkable sentence in a manuscript dedicated to the Danish king is quoted here, since it is as timely now as it was then:

The heart has been considered the seat of natural warmth, as the throne of the soul, and even as the soul itself. Some have greeted the heart as the sun, others as the king, but if you examine it more closely, one finds it to be nothing more than muscle.

Those who are shocked by cardiac xenografts or those who are awed by the mystique of heart transplantation should remember this sentence of Stensen's.

However, it was in Leyden that he described the heart of an embryo with the cardiac malformation entitled, *"Stenonis, N: Embryo monstro affinis Parisiis dissectus, 1665. Acta Medica et Philosophica Hafniensia 1:200–203, 1673."* This refers to the first volume of Thomas Bartholin's *Acta Medica.* I was made aware of this by, Albert Gjedde, Professor of Physiology in Copenhagen, who informed me that the *Acta Medica et Philosophica Hafniensia* was the first regularly published medical journal in the world, later revived as *Nordisk Medicinist Archiv.* It was translated from Latin into German by G. Scherz, a Jesuit who became expert on Stenoniana, and into Danish by E. Warburg in the *Nordisk Medicine* in December 1942; into English by F.A. Willius, and published in the *Cardiac Clinic CXXIV,* in the staff meetings of the Mayo Clinic in 1948. Obviously Stensen's embryo had other malformations, such as cleft palate, which the mother ascribed to "her craving for rabbit meat." The fetus was also that of a hermaphrodite. But it was the heart that intrigued Stensen:

It became clear to me that the canal which leads from the pulmonary artery to the aorta, and which is clearly visible in every embryo, was completely absent. When I opened the right ventricle, the probe introduced into the right ventricle . . . could be advanced directly into the aorta. The right ventricle here has three openings, one from the atrium, two into the large arteries. The aorta has a common origin from both ventricles . . . .

He also clearly described the course of blood from the right ventricle into both the pulmonary artery and the aorta.

In 1666, Stensen left Paris for Florence and became connected with the Hospital of Santa Maria Nuova and converted to Catholicism. Shortly afterwards he was offered a position by the Danish king. In 1672, Stensen returned to Copenhagen. He again became involved in controversies (what creative individual does not?) with the Rector of the University. He resigned his position in 1674 and returned to Florence, where he took charge of the education of one of the Medicis, the son of the Grand Duke Cosimo III. In 1675, Stensen became a priest and soon afterwards a bishop. After several years of restless peregrinations, he died in northern Germany in 1686. The Grand Duke of Tuscany sent for his body and he was buried in Florence, entombed with the Grand Dukes in St. Lorenzo. Thus ends one of the most remarkable careers of an early pediatric cardiopathologist. An ingenious inventor (he was also a pioneer geologist), who was caught in the dangerous web spun in the twilight between Renaissance and Baroque, he was a victim of his own restless genius and of his personal drive to reconcile it with the world about him.

The descriptive period of pathological anatomy in congenital heart disease did not end with the seventeenth century. Rather, within our own time and generation, descriptive pathology of congenital heart disease has continued to flourish. Surgeons have been able to correct many of the hitherto inaccessible malformations, and an exact knowledge of the nature of these malformations is an absolute prerequisite for corrective surgery. Maude Abbott, Richard Van Praagh, and Jesse Edwards are just a few of those who, working with the cardiac surgeons, have accurately defined the anatomy of unusual cardiac malformations.

As mentioned previously the second overlapping phase of the development in congenital heart disease is concerned with the physiological pattern of the malformation. These studies are relatively recent, and credit for their initiation must go to a large extent to

Alfred Blalock of Johns Hopkins Hospital. It was he who sparked the organization of a laboratory almost exclusively devoted to this field. He was a "natural" to show interest in physiopathology. Years of physiological research at Vanderbilt, some of it in cooperation with Tinsley Harrison, had prepared him for this work. After I had been discharged from the Army Medical Corps, I started in this laboratory, initiated by Blalock in 1945. The years at Hopkins were full of excitement and discovery. Everything in this field was new. The diagnosis and nature of pulmonary hypertension, of transposition of the great vessels, the tetralogy of Fallot, and so on were all challenging subjects. At that time, the laboratories at Bellevue with Cournand, at the Brigham with Dexter, and at Emory with Warren and Stead were the pioneering institutions. It must be remembered that Blalock was particularly proud of his work on shock and justifiably so. As Ravitch wrote, "His own evaluation, with which history will agree, is that that work in which he stressed importance of fluid lack and replacement in shock, was his greatest scientific contribution."

What impressed me most was his disregard for the yield of practical results from our laboratory. He was happy to have us publish purely physiological data and was most pleased when we published data on mechanism of adjustments of cyanotic children to hypoxia. The fact that catheterization of the heart, a relatively new tool, also was used by us for diagnostic purposes was of secondary importance. These patients gave us as an opportunity to study the effects of anoxia, of increased pulmonary flow, or of large intracardiac shunts. It was essential for our understanding to outline diagrammatically the circulatory pattern of each malformation. This is how we came to describe for the first time a particular type of partial transposition of the great vessels, with the pulmonary artery "overriding both ventricles" and the aorta transposed with its origin from the right ventricle.[1] Taussig clinically had encountered the puzzling picture of this malformation, and the combined clinical and physiopathological description made this malformation a clinical and pathological entity. I am grateful to Maurice Lev, who named this malformation the Taussig-Bing heart, which assured me a degree of precarious immortality.[2]

Like most great men, Blalock was a complicated personality. To those who did not know him well, he was an urbane Southern gentleman. Had he been just that he could not have accomplished what he set out to do. He was an extremely hard working and dedicated surgeon who expected to be followed and listened to. He was extremely fair, but expected as much hard work from others as he did from himself. For ten years before I went to Baltimore, I had worked with Alexis Carrel at the Rockefeller Institute. No two people could have been more different: the Frenchman, Alexis Carrel, always scintillating, always full of ideas; and the gentleman from Georgia, Alfred Blalock, systematic and steady. Both had one thing in common: they were hard as rock when it came to self-discipline, and this they expected from others.

Right heart catheterization was the beginning of accurate diagnosis of congenital heart disease. Yet, I look back with astonishment and envy at some cardiologists who relied on the stethoscope and the fluoroscope and could accomplish great feats of diagnostic skill with these simple tools, together with clinical divinations. Inevitably, our exact sister science, physics, had to lend a helping hand. With that help, diagnosis of congenital heart disease, along with most of cardiology, has utilized noninvasive procedures (e.g., echocardiography and nuclear magnetic resonance imaging). How much this latter technique will contribute to the diagnosis of congenital heart disease is uncertain. Without question the future lies in noninvasive techniques.

What about surgical treatment? This book testifies to its advance. What brought about this tremendous acceleration of cardiac surgery? Foremost, the work of John Gibbon, who spent nineteen years developing the pump oxygenator to a practical reality, despite the lack of encouragement of the "men of measured mean," the Geheim-räte. Gibbon had no government fund to help him along, and there was no Presidential Advisory Board to speed his progress. As for the shunt operation for the tetralogy of Fallot, Blalock was a natural for its initiation. Together with Levi (Leeds) he had, from purely physiological considerations, carried out this shunt operation on dogs at Vanderbilt to see whether or not an increase in pulmonary blood flow would result in an elevation in pulmonary artery pressure. What this operation accomplished was not (as some believed) the increase in "effective pulmonary blood flow" (blood effectively oxygenated in the lungs).

Why did I leave this field of plenty at the Johns Hopkins Hospital to exile myself to the provinces? This was no exile! The provinces were the University of Alabama, in which Tinsley Harrison played a vital and exciting role. My main reason was that I had by chance pushed the catheter into the coronary sinus: this opened a whole new field, that of cardiac metabolism. It also seemed to me that the verdant meadows of congenital heart disease had been thoroughly grazed of apparent physiological pasture. There remained plenty to do diagnostically, but the yield in physiological and fundamental knowledge showed diminishing returns. I was determined to carry out these new studies on cardiac metabolism. Blalock apparently was not pleased by my diversion into fields so completely alien from his main interest. However, three years later (in 1956), just before I was to give a Harvey Lecture in New York, I received from Alfred Blalock a telegram of congratulations which I treasure.

Much has happened in the field of congenital heart disease since then. We have a new subspecialty, pediatric cardiology. We have magnificently equipped diagnostic laboratories with expensive electronic equipment that makes our laboratory at Johns Hopkins in the early 1940s look like an alchemist's shop. The emphasis in cardiac surgery has shifted to the coronaries, and in the field of congenital heart disease, nothing but radical repair will do.

Obvious to all of us is the fact that the history of surgery for congenital heart disease is but a prelude to the future.

References

1. Taussig HB, Bing RJ: Complete transposition of the aorta and a levoposition of the pulmonary artery. *Am Heart J* 37:551, 1949
2. Lev M, Rimoldi HJA, Eckner FAO, Melhuish BB, Heng CCL, Paul MH: The Taussig-Bing heart. Qualitative and quantitative anatomy. *Arch Pathol* 81:24–35, 1966.

Section II
Left Heart Obstructive Lesions

As doctors we should sometimes think not only about our dexterity and our cleverness in diagnosis, but what sort of human beings we are going to produce and what sort of family will remain when you have done your best and when you have done your worst.

Jane Somerville, M.D.
Obstructive Lesions of the Right Heart

Introduction

Masato Takahashi, M.D.

Obstruction of the left ventricular outflow tract encompasses a wide spectrum both in anatomy and physiology. This section begins with a chapter by Dr. Richard Van Praagh and coauthors describing anatomic variations in congenital valvar, subvalvar, and supravalvar aortic stenosis. The authors put forth important anatomic features common in each category of lesions, and then develop the discussion toward description of variations on the theme. One gets a clear mental image of functional anatomy of the aortic valve as the authors graphically describe commissures and valve leaflets.

The second chapter by Dr. Alan Lewis lays physiologic foundations for understanding left heart obstructive lesions by developing the concepts of ventricular wall stress, determinants of myocardial oxygen consumption, and supply/demand ratio. He then shows various adaptive changes in response to the outflow obstruction, impact of growth, and special problems of newborn myocardium.

Dr. Winfield Wells' chapter gives a profile of surgical experience with congenital aortic stenosis with a large number of patients over a long span of time and brings to focus a number of problems, including late deaths due to bacterial endocarditis, and needs for reoperation due to restenosis, especially in patients with multilevel obstructions. He points out that the incidence of surgically induced aortic regurgitation may be kept low, thus minimizing the need for prosthetic valves.

Dr. Gordon Danielson describes the Mayo Clinic experiences in various types of aortic valve prostheses in a historical perspective. His discussion is extended to include the use of apical conduits.

Dr. Albert Pacifico tackles the challenging problem of enlarging the small aortic annulus. He graphically describes the posterior and anterior approaches. He also discusses in sufficient detail the techniques of harvesting, storage, and implanting human aortic valve homografts.

11

Discussion of left heart obstructive lesions is not complete without mentioning the hypoplastic left heart syndrome, the severest and most challenging among this subset of cardiac lesions. In a spirit of the surgical frontier, Dr. Leonard Bailey gives an account of his team efforts in animal research and clinical trial of cardiac xenograft transplant.

CHAPTER 2

Anatomic Variations in Congenital Valvar, Subvalvar, and Supravalvar Aortic Stenosis: A Study of 64 Postmortem Cases

Richard Van Praagh, M.D., Antonio Baño-Rodrigo, M.D., Aram Smolinsky, M.D., Thomas J. Schuetz, B.Sc., Donald C. Fyler, M.D., Stella Van Praagh, M.D.*

What is congenital aortic stenosis from the standpoint of pathological anatomy? In an effort to answer this question, a study was undertaken of all cases in the Cardiac Registry of the Boston Children's Hospital in which the primary diagnosis was congenital aortic stenosis.[1]

Findings

Congenital aortic stenosis was the primary diagnosis in 64 of the 2,492 autopsied cases now in the Cardiac Registry (2.6%). Male/female ratio was 47/16 (2.9/1), the sex being unknown in one patient. Males thus accounted for 75% of this postmortem series. The median age at death was 3.5 months, ranging from 1.4 hours to 31$\frac{4}{12}$ years.

Anatomical Types

The anatomical types of congenital aortic stenosis that were found in this study of 64 postmortem cases are summarized in Table I.

---

*This presentation is based on a paper that has been submitted for publication to the *American Journal of Cardiology*.

Table I
Anatomic Types of Congenital Aortic Stenosis
N = 64

Salient Anatomic Features	No of Cases	Percentage of Series*
I. Valvar	51	80
Tricuspid aortic valve	2	3
Bicuspid aortic valve	14	22
Unicuspid aortic valve	34	53
Acuspid aortic valve	1	2
II. Subvalvar		
Fibrous	7	11
III. Supravalvar	6	9

*Percentages rounded off to the nearest whole number.

I. Valvar

Valvar congenital aortic stenosis was the most frequent type of congenital aortic stenosis found in this study (51 cases, 80% of the series, Table 1).

Valvar congenital aortic stenosis was found to be tricuspid in only two cases (3% of the series as a whole), bicuspid in 14 cases (22%), unicuspid in 34 cases (53%), and acuspid in one patient (2% of the series).

In valvar congenital aortic stenosis (AS), it was found that:

1. the number of functional leaflets equalled the number of effective (normally developed and underdeveloped) commissures; or, expressed differently,
2. the number of functional leaflets equalled 3 minus the number of virtually absent commissures. For example, when one commissure was absent, the number of functional leaflets equalled 3 minus 1, i.e., 2. When two commissures were absent, the number of functional leaflets equalled 3 minus 2, i.e., 1.

In so-called bicuspid aortic valve (AoV) and unicuspid AoV, all three leaflets typically were found to be present, but with essential absence of one or two commissures—in functionally bicuspid and functionally unicuspid AoV, respectively.

It was observed that, accurately speaking, a bicuspid AoV is a *bicommissural* AoV and a unicuspid AoV is a *unicommissural* AoV.

The function of the commissures of the AoV appeared to be the following:

1. to divide the aortic valve leaflet substance into separate leaflets;
2. to support the aortic valve leaflets.

In Figure 1, the left coronary/noncoronary (LC/NC) commissure is well developed, dividing the LC leaflet from the NC leaflet. However, the right coronary/noncoronary (RC/NC) commissure is absent; hence the RC and NC leaflets are continuous. The RC/LC commissure is rudimentary; consequently the RC and LC leaflets also are continuous. Thus, the NC, RC, and LC leaflets all are continuous, being divided only by the LC/NC commissure, resulting in a so-called unicuspid (i.e., unicommissural) AoV (Fig. 1). It is also noteworthy that the AoV leaflet tissue is thick and has gelatinous and myxomatous consistency, that the orifice of the AoV is markedly reduced in size, and that the aortic annulus is smaller than normal. Hence, we found that valvar congenital aortic stenosis typically displays three different kinds of abnormality: (1) commissural absence or deficiency, (2) leaflet thickening, and (3) annular smallness (hypoplasia). These three different but coexisting kinds of valvar pathology contributed to reduction of the aortic orifice, resulting in aortic valvar stenosis.

When an aortic commissure was absent—typically the RC/NC—the unsupported aortic leaflets tended to *prolapse downward*, filling and largely occluding the left ventricular outflow tract (Fig. 2). In such hearts, it was difficult to push one's index finger from the left ventricle (LV) into the ascending aorta (Ao) because the downwardly prolapsed aortic valve leaflet tissue (RC and NC) was very fibrous, firm, and uncompliant (Fig. 2). This remarkably firm leaflet tissue also was the site of *calcification* and *bacterial endocarditis* (Fig. 3).

Congenital aortic valvar stenosis was found to be very different from acquired aortic valvar stenosis. In congenital AS, the leaflets are *not fused* (as they are in chronic rheumatic aortic stenosis). Instead, in congenital AS, the leaflets are *unseparated* due to commissural rudi-

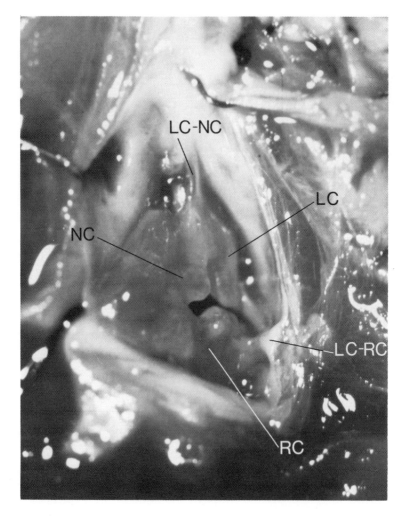

Figure 1. Unicuspid (unicommissural) aortic valve resulting in severe congenital aortic stenosis. Only the left coronary-noncoronary commissure (LC-NC) is well developed. The left coronary-right coronary commissure (LC-RC) is rudimentary. The right coronary-noncoronary commissure (RC-NC) is absent. All three leaflets (LC, RC and NC) are present in this so-called unicuspid valve, which really is unicommissural, i.e., only one well-developed commissure, which almost always is the LC-NC. The leaflets are thick and myxomatous and the annulus is small. (Premature 19-hour-old male born following a 34-week gestation.)

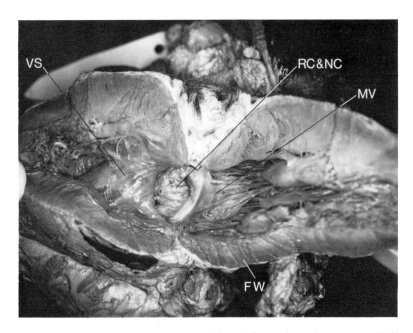

Figure 2. *Bicuspid aortic valve viewed from below. The right coronary (RC) and noncoronary (NC) leaflets are continuous (undivided) because the RC-NC commissure is rudimentary. The elongated and markedly thickened right coronary plus noncoronary leaflet (RC & NC) has prolapsed downward, almost totally occluding the left ventricular outflow tract between the anterior leaflet of the mitral valve (MV) and the ventricular septum (VS). FW = free wall. (A 24 ⁴/₁₂-year-old man who died when his car struck a hydrant, resulting in multiple transmural aortic and right atrial lacerations. Ventricular arrhythmia may have caused accident; he may have died before the accident occurred.)*

mentary development or absence (Fig. 4). The other very prominent pathological feature of congenital AS is the marked leaflet *thickening* (Fig. 5).

The foregoing are the general pathological anatomic features of valvar congenital aortic stenosis. Now we will consider the findings in the various anatomical subsets of valvar congenital aortic stenosis in somewhat greater detail.

1. Tricuspid Valvar Congenital Aortic Stenosis

Only two patients (Table I), an 8.5-month-old boy and a 26-year-old man, had valvar AS with a tricuspid AoV.

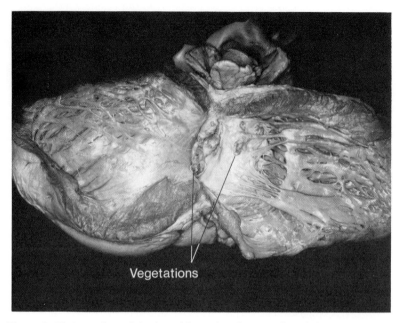

Vegetations

Figure 3. *Unicommissural (unicuspid) aortic valve seen from below. Only the LC-NC commissure was well developed, the other two being absent. The thick fibrous leaflet tissue herniated down into the LV outflow tract, largely occluding it. Note that on these prolapsing aortic valvar "hemorrhoids" there are multiple vegetations with one of the anterior leaflets of the mitral valve.*

The 8.5-month-old male (A76-93) had what we believe to be a *rare combination* of (1) preductal coarctation of the aorta, (2) valvar congenital aortic stenosis, and (3) valvar congenital pulmonary stenosis (PS). The valvar AS and the coexisting valvar PS were severe. Both the aortic and the pulmonary valves were tricuspid (tricommissural). Both the aortic and the pulmonary leaflets displayed marked myxomatous and fibrous thickening. There was moderate peripheral pulmonary stenosis at the proximal branching of the right pulmonary artery, and biventricular hypertrophy was massive.

2. Bicuspid Valvar Congenital Aortic Stenosis

Bicuspid valvar congenital aortic stenosis was the second most common form of AS encountered in this postmortem series (22%, Table I). *The state of the aortic commissures* was as follows:

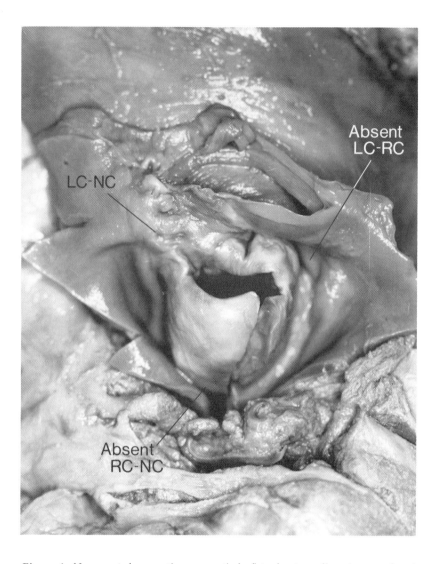

Figure 4. *Unseparated or continuous aortic leaflets due to rudimentary or absent commissures. Only the left coronary-noncoronary commissure (LC-NC) is well developed, the left coronary-right coronary (LC-RC) and the right coronary-noncoronary (RC-NC) commissures being absent in this typical uni-commissural (functionally unicuspid) valve. (A 13⁷/₁₂-year-old boy who died intraoperatively in 1956 and whose heart weighed 720 g, 120 g being normal.)*

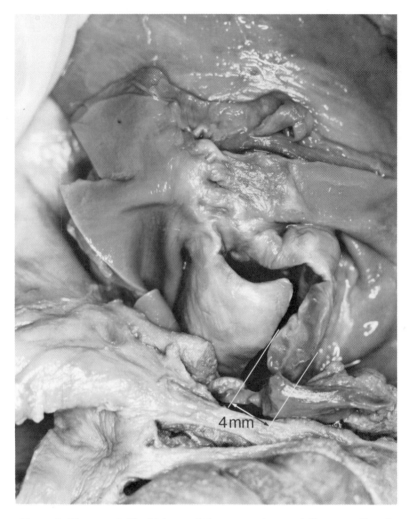

Figure 5. *The remarkable thickness of the myxomatous and fibrous aortic valve leaflet tissue is noteworthy (4 mm). (Same case as Fig. 4.)*

1. the RC/NC commissure was rudimentary (a raphé), the RC/LC commissure was underdeveloped, and the LC/NC commissure was well developed in 7 of these 14 cases (50%);

2. the RC/NC commissure was rudimentary, the other two commissures were well developed in 4 of 14 cases (29%); and
3. the RC/LC commissure was rudimentary, the other two were well developed in 3 of 14 cases (21%).

In the foregoing data, it is noteworthy that the RC/NC commissure was by far the most often absent or rudimentary (79%), and that the LC/NC commissure always was well developed.

Male/female ratio was 11/3 (3.7/1).

The median age at death in this autopsied subgroup was 10 months, ranging from 10 days to 19 years. These ages at death do not necessarily reflect the natural history of bicuspid valvar congenital AS, because 8 of these 14 deaths (57%) occurred postoperatively. *Thick, myxomatous, fibrous aortic leaflets* occurred in all. *Endocardial fibroelastosis* (EFE) of the left ventricle was found in two of these 14 patients (14%).

In these 14 cases, there was one patient (7%) with each of the following: congenital mitral stenosis (arcade), congenital mitral regurgitation, postductal coarctation of the aorta, sudden unexpected death, left ventricular myocardial infarction, sepsis, bacterial endarteritis, and acute bronchopneumonia.

3. Unicuspid Valvar Congenital Aortic Stenosis

This was by far the most common form of congenital AS found in this postmortem series (53%, Table I) (Fig. 1).

The *only well-developed commissure*, i.e., of normal height, was:

1. LC/NC in 32/34 cases (94%);
2. RC/NC in 1/34 cases (3%); and
3. RC/LC in 1/34 cases (3%).

The male sex predominance was again found in this group: males/females = 26/7 (3.7/1), the sex being unknown in one case.

The *ages at death* in these 34 autopsied cases were: median, 7 days and range from 1.5 hours to $24^{4}/_{12}$ years. Of these 34 patients, 14 died intraoperatively or postoperatively (41%).

EFE of the LV (Fig. 6) was found in 26 of these 34 cases of

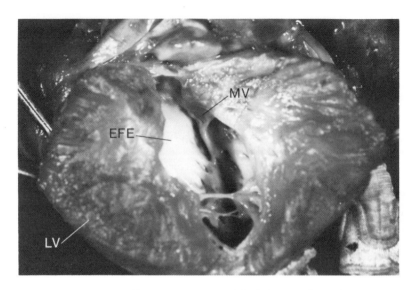

Figure 6. *Endocardial fibroelastosis (EFE) of the left ventricle (LV) occurred in 76% of cases with unicuspid (unicommissural) congenital aortic stenosis. Note the small-chambered LV cavity, the remarkably thick LV free wall (20–25 mm), the pearly white LV septal surface, the hypoplasia (stenosis) of the mitral valve (MV), and the hypoplasia of the papillary muscles. (Two-month-old female.)*

unicuspid (unicommissural) valvar congenital aortic stenosis (76%), all had a patent mitral valve and an intact ventricular septum.

Marked thickening of the aortic leaflet tissue was present in all.

Mitral hypoplasia was found in 16 of these 34 cases (47%).

Sudden unexpected death occurred in 5 of these patients (15%).

Multiple congenital anomalies were found in 3 of these 34 cases (8.9%).

Myocardial infarction was found in 2 of the 34 (6%), involving the left ventricle in one and the right ventricle in the other.

Premature closure of the foramen ovale was observed in 1 of the 34 patients (3%), a male who died at 1.5 hours of age. Septum primum (the flap valve of the foramen ovale) displayed no ostium secundum or other opening.

A rare form of parachute mitral valve (MV) was found in 1 of these 34 cases. All of the chordae tendineae of the mitral valve inserted into the anterolateral papillary muscle group of the left ventricle, the posteromedial papillary muscle group being absent. In parachute

MV, it typically is the anterolateral papillary muscle group that is absent—except with common AV canal,[2] in which the posteromedial papillary muscle group can be absent as in this case. However, our patient with this rare form of parachute MV (with absent posteromedial papillary muscle group) did not have common AV canal.

Congenital mitral regurgitation occurred in 3 of these 34 cases (8.9%). One of these patients had absence of the anterolateral papillary muscle group, but without parachute mitral valve because the anterolateral mitral chordae inserted directly into the left ventricular free wall.

One patient had each of the following: valvar pulmonary stenosis, muscular ventricular septal defect, absence of septum primum, and aberrant origin of left coronary artery from the interior surface of the left pulmonary artery.

4. Acuspid Valvar Congenital Aortic Stenosis

One patient, a 5-month-old girl, had no well formed aortic leaflets, just masses of firm, myxomatous, fibrous tissue about the aortic annulus. The RC/NC and RC/LC commissures were rudimentary (raphae only) while the LC/NC was absent (not even a raphe being found). Diffuse EFE of the LV and massive left ventricular hypertrophy and enlargement were present.

The *state of the aortic commissures* in valvar congenital aortic stenosis is summarized in Table II.

II. Subvalvar

Subaortic fibrous stenosis occurred in 7 of these 64 autopsied cases of congenital aortic stenosis (11%, Table I). Although the male predominance continued with males/females = 5/2 (2.5/1), the ages at death were very much older than in valvar aortic stenosis: median = 13 years, range = 5.5 months to $27^{10}/_{12}$ years. Of these 7 patients, 4 died postoperatively (57%).

What is *congenital fibrous subaortic stenosis*? In this study it was found to be:

1. a discrete fibrous ring in 5 of 7 cases (71%) (Fig. 7); and

Table II
State of the Commissures in Valvar Congenital Aortic Stenosis
N = 51

	RC/NC			RC/LC			LC/NC		
	+	−	0	+	−	0	+	−	0
Tricuspid AoV, N = 2	2			2			2		
Bicuspid AoV, N = 14	3		11	4	7	3	14		
Unicuspid AoV, N = 34	1		33	1		33	32		2
Acuspid AoV, N = 1			1			1			1

AoV, aortic value; N, number; RC/NC, right coronary/noncoronary commissure; RC/LC, right coronary/left coronary commissure; LC/NC, left coronary/noncoronary commissure; +, well developed; −, underdeveloped; 0, absent or rudimentary.

2. an obstructive anterior leaflet of the mitral valve in 2 of 7 cases (29%) (Fig. 8).
3. *Endocardial fibroelastosis* occurred in none of these cases of subaortic congenital fibrous stenosis.
4. *Multiple congenital anomalies* were found in two.
5. Stenosis at all three levels—subvalvar, valvar, and supravalvar—occurred in one patient, a $27^{10}/_{12}$-year-old man.
6. *Mild thickening of the aortic valve leaflets* was found in all cases of subaortic stenosis.

III. Supravalvar

Supravalvar congenital aortic stenosis (Fig. 9) occurred in 6 of these 64 autopsied cases (9%, Table I). Neither sex predominated, males/females = 3/3 (1/1). The median age at death was 18.75 years, the range being from 6 months to 31.3 years. Of these six patients, four died postoperatively (67%). Hence, these ages at death do not reflect the natural history of supravalvar aortic stenosis. Nonetheless, it is noteworthy in Table III that supravalvar aortic stenosis was the type of congenital AS that had by far the oldest median age at death (18.75 years) and the oldest patient in this series, a $31^{4}/_{12}$-year-old woman.

The salient finding in this group of supravalvar congenital aortic stenosis was that *Williams' syndrome* is a *generalized arteriopathy*. Not

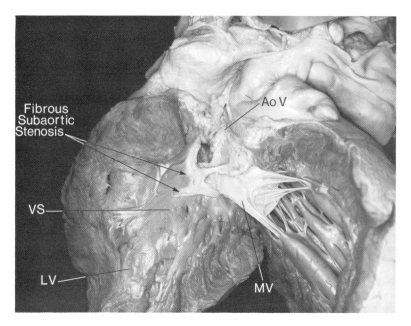

Figure 7. *Fibrous subaortic stenosis. The thickened and heaped up fibrous tissue extends from the anterior leaflet of the mitral valve (MV) over onto the left ventricular septal surface (VS). This fibrous tissue is often continuous with the leaflets of the aortic valve (AoV) and may overlie the membranous septum and the conduction system. (13¹¹/₁₂-year-old male who died from acute promyelocytic leukemia.)*

only was the immediately supravalvar aortic region characterized by marked aortic thickening, but so too were the ascending aorta, the transverse aortic arch, and the isthmus (Fig. 9B). In one patient, even the coronary arteries displayed striking mural thickening with luminal narrowing. One patient, a 12-year-old boy, had a narrowed aortic isthmus where he developed a jet lesion, and then a mycotic aneurysm, which ruptured into the upper lobe of the left lung.

Congenital aortic valvar stenosis was found in three of these six cases, two having markedly thickened tricuspid aortic valves and one having a thickened bicuspid aortic valve with an underdeveloped RC/NC commissure.

Congenital pulmonary valvar stenosis coexisted in two patients.

Hypotension with sedation during cardiac catheterization appeared to have contributed to the death of a 6-month-old girl with typical

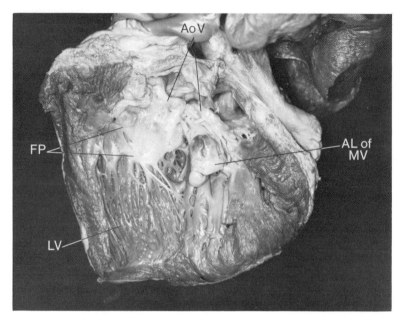

Figure 8. Severe subaortic stenosis produced by the anterior leaflet of the mitral valve (AL of MV), which is thickened, myxomatous, fibrous, and involved by blood cysts. Opposite the AL of MV, there is a prominent fibrous plaque (FP) on the left ventricular (LV) septal surface below the aortic valve (AoV). The AL of MV and the FP almost totally occlude the LV outflow tract. The FP is regarded as a jet lesion and impact lesion related to the AL of MV. (A 5²/₁₂-year-old boy with dysmorphic facies, multiple congenital anomalies, and polyvalvular disease with similar changes of tricuspid valve.)

Williams' syndrome.[3] In addition to supravalvar aortic stenosis and pulmonary valvar stenosis, autopsy revealed generalized arteriopathy with marked thickening of the aortic and pulmonary walls. The coronary arteries were ropelike with considerable mural thickening and luminal narrowing. Concentric left ventricular hypertrophy was massive (11 mm in thickness) and moderate right ventricular hypertrophy also was present.

A small aortic annulus in Williams' syndrome led to surgical difficulties in a 31⁴/₁₂-year-old woman. In order to enlarge the aortic annulus, an incision was carried into the anterior mitral leaflet. Subsequently, this part of the repair broke down, requiring mitral valve, replacement, which was complicated by chronic perivalvular leak, leading to death from congestive heart failure.

Aortic prosthetic valve failure led to the death of a 24-year-old man with Williams' syndrome. The occluder of his #21 Bjork–Shiley prosthesis became immobilized by pannus formation after six years, resulting in marked aortic prosthetic valvar stenosis.

Immobilization of the noncoronary leaflet of the aortic valve against a Dacron gusset placed into the noncoronary sinus of Valsalva led to severe aortic regurgitation and death in a 20³/₁₂-year-old man. At autopsy, the immobilized noncoronary aortic leaflet was stone-like and fused with the Dacron gusset.

Discussion

Congenital aortic stenosis is at least three different diseases:

1. Usually, it was a *valvar* anomaly, as in 80% of this autopsied series (Table I).
2. Occasionally, it was a *subvalvular* fibrous obstruction, as in 11% of this series (Table I). We think that fibrous subaortic stenosis represents residual atrioventricular canal endocardial cushion tissue, this subaortic fibrous tissue being closely related to the tissue of the anterior leaflet of the mitral valve.
3. The least frequent form of congenital aortic stenosis in this series (11%, Table I) was supravalvar obstruction, which we think essentially is a diffuse arteriopathy.

Commissurotomy does not apply to congenital aortic stenosis (AS) in the same way that it applies to acquired (e.g., rheumatic) AS, because in congenital AS, the aortic leaflets are not fused. Instead, they are *unseparated* and *unsupported* because of failure of commissure formation. Hence, commissurotomy at the site of an absent or deficient commissure runs the risk of producing two flail aortic leaflets (because of lack of commissural support).[4] Nonetheless, because of the thick, myxomatous, fibrous leaflet tissue, it is our impression that a relatively small aortic *valvotomy* (not necessarily commissurotomy), or aortic valve tearing with a balloon,[5] may have some beneficial effect in the treatment of severe valvar congenital

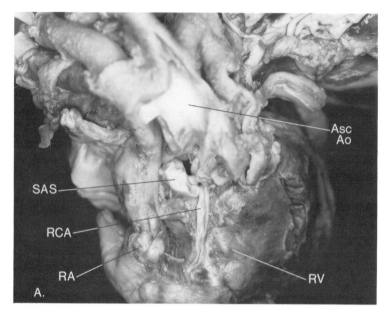

Figure 9A. *Williams' syndrome of supravalvar aortic stenosis and general-ized arteriopathy. View of aortic root. Note that the aortic root is markedly thickened immediately above the right coronary artery (RCA), resulting in supravalvar aortic stenosis. The coronary arteries are ropelike with thick walls and small lumina, but without thrombi. (A 6-month-old female who died in the Cardiac Catherterization laboratory as a result of irreversible systemic hypotension following routine sedation. We speculate that ketamine anesthesia, which produces systemic hypertension, may be helpful in this kind of situation. Hypotension, with this kind of generalized and restrictive arteriopathy, must be avoided if possible.)*

aortic stenosis. It seems that the uncompliant nature of the aortic leaflets makes the risk of postoperative aortic insufficiency much less than would be the case if the consistency of the aortic leaflets were normal. This is one of the reasons why aortic valvotomy or balloon tearing virtually anywhere appears to be a therapeutically beneficial procedure. Since resistance varies inversely as the fourth power of the radius (Poiseuille's law), even small increases in the radius of the aortic orifice can have relatively large effects in lowering the resistance offered by a stenotic aortic valve.

The *ages at death* in this postmortem series (Table III) do not necessarily reflect the natural history of congenital aortic stenosis

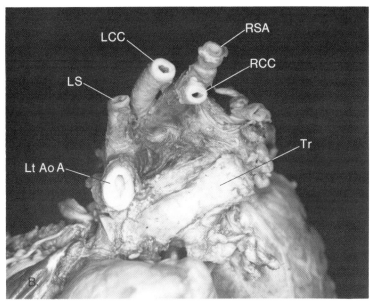

Figure 9B. *View of transected brachiocephalic arteries and left aortic arch (Lt AoA). Note that the walls of the right common carotid artery (RCC), left common carotid artery (LCC), and the aortic arch (Lt AoA) are remarkably thickened. A preductal coarctation of the aorta was almost produced by the marked thickening of the aortic wall. Asc Ao, ascending aorta; LS, left subclavian artery; RA, right atrium; RSA, right subclavian artery; RV, right ventricle; Tr, trachea.*

because many of these patients died postoperatively (see Findings). Also, the findings presented in this series do not reflect the surgical mortality rate at our hospital, because these findings are based on postmortem cases only. Nonetheless, assuming that these patients were operated on when their clinical condition demanded it, the median ages of death (Table III) suggest that supravalvar aortic stenosis (Williams' syndrome) has the best natural history (median age at death, 18.75 years, Table III). Subvalvar fibrous aortic stenosis appears to have the second best natural history (median age at death, 13 years, Table III). Valvar aortic stenosis seems to have the least favorable natural history (Table III), cases with a unicuspid (unicommissural) aortic valve (median age at death, 7 days, Table III) being the worst form, and cases with a bicuspid

Table III
Ages at Death in Congenital Aortic Stenosis

Types of Aortic Stenosis	Median	Range
I. Valvar		
Tricuspid aortic valve	*	8.5 mos–26 yrs
Bicuspid aortic valve	10 mos	10 days–19 yrs
Unicuspid aortic valve	7 days	1.4 hrs–24$^{4}/_{12}$ yrs
Acuspid aortic valve	**	5 mos–
II. Subvalvar		
Fibrous	13 yrs	5.5 mos–27$^{10}/_{12}$ yrs
III. Supravalvar	18.75 yrs	6 mos–31$^{4}/_{12}$ yrs

*Only two cases, therefore median not given.
**Only one case, therefore median not given.

aortic valve (median age at death, 10 months, Table III) being somewhat better.

The *frequency of endocardial fibroelastosis* (EFE) was 76% in patients with a unicuspid aortic valve and 14% in patients with a bicuspid aortic valve, again supporting the concept that, in general, unicuspid AS is the worst form.

What does left ventricular EFE mean? Why do we regard left ventricular EFE as an index of severity of congenital aortic valvar stenosis? Because EFE tends to be associated only with the most severely stenotic cases. When the aortic stenosis is less severe, the incidence of left ventricular EFE declines sharply. EFE of the left ventricle (LV) is virtually always present with aortic atresia if the mitral valve is patent and if the ventricular septum is intact; but if a sizable ventricular septal defect (VSD) coexists with aortic atresia, then EFE of the LV is never present, in our experience. If mitral atresia coexists with aortic atresia, then the small LV never has EFE.

Consequently, when LV outflow tract obstruction (stenosis or atresia) is present, left ventricular EFE appears to represent an old global subendocardial myocardial infarction with replacement fibrosis. Our hypothesis is that if the LV pressure in diastole remains above the coronary perfusion pressure in the subendocardial layer during diastole, then diffuse left ventricular subendocardial ischemic necrosis, followed by fibrosis, will occur. This happens only in the most severe cases of LV outflow tract obstruction. Our hypothesis is that when it is possible for the LV diastolic pressure to drop below that of the coronary diastolic pressure, then subendocardial perfusion is adequate and so-called EFE does not occur. Factors favoring the absence of EFE are anything that permits the LV diastolic pressure to fall—such as a decompressing VSD, or not extremely severe aortic stenosis.

This kind of EFE is known as *secondary EFE*, meaning that the EFE is secondary (to severe LV outflow tract obstruction, as above). There is another kind of EFE which is more rare, known as *Primary EFE*, meaning that the EFE is not secondary to LV outflow tract obstruction.

Consequently, the much higher frequency of secondary EFE in unicuspid aortic stenosis (76%) than in bicuspid aortic stenosis (14%) is a statistically significant difference (p<0.0005), which we think supports the concept that unicuspid aortic stenosis tends to be more severe than does bicuspid aortic stenosis.

It must be remembered that although statistical data are true in general, they do not necessarily apply to an individual case. For example, fibrous subaortic stenosis typically is not extremely severe and usually lacks EFE (see Findings). Rarely, however, fibrous subaortic stenosis can be of profound severity (Figs. 10-12),[6] and when mitral regurgitation is absent, severe EFE can coexist (Fig. 12).[6] In all forms of congenital aortic stenosis, the range—on both sides of the median age at death—was very large (Table III).

Regarding frequency, congenital AS accounts for 2.6% of all cases in the Cardiac Registry of the Boston Children's Hospital. But since these are postmortem statistics, they do not bear any necessary relationship to what is happening in the real world. In an effort to correct this deficiency, we have sought relevant comparable data from the New England Regional Infant Cardiac Program (RICP).[7] In the first year of life, congenital AS was diagnosed in 1.9% of patients seen (45 of 2,381 infants with congenital heart disease). Of these 45 infants with congenital AS, 51% died in the first year of life. Valvar AS was present in 41 (91%), subvalvar stenosis in one (2%), and supravalvar AS in 3 (7%). More than 80% were male.

Although the RICP frequency of congenital AS in living patients during the first year of life (1.9%) was lower than the total pathology frequency (2.6%), the frequency of congenital AS climbed sharply in older age groups: 0–5 years, 3%; 5–10 years, 8%; 10–15 years, 12%; 15–20 years, 17%; 20–25 years, 17%; and 25–60 years, 16%. The data under one year of age were derived from the RICP,[7] while the data

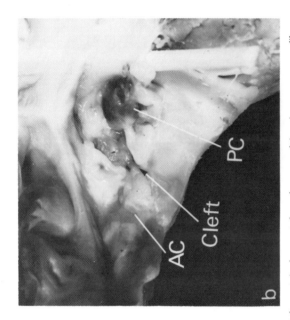

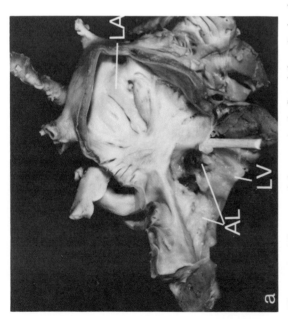

Figure 10. Adherence of the anterior leaflet of the mitral valve to the left ventricular septal surface, resulting in very severe fibrous subaortic stenosis and free mitral regurgitation. *a*, left lateral view of opened left atrium (LA), mitral valve, and left ventricle (LV), the apex of which was amputated at autopsy. *b*, close-up view of anterior leaflet of mitral valve. In *a*, the anterior leaflet (AL) of the mitral valve is tightly adherent to the left ventricular (LV) septal surface. Subaortic fibrous stenosis is very marked, the only outlet from the LV demonstrated by a small wooden probe. Since the fibrous tissue that should have formed the anterior leaflet of the mitral valve is plastered against the LV septal surface, producing severe fibrous subaortic stenosis, there is no functional anterior leaflet of the mitral valve; hence, there was free mitral regurgitation into the hypertrophied and enlarged LA. In *b*, the anterior cushion (AC) and posterior cushion (PC) components of what should have been the anterior leaflet of the mitral valve, and the cleft between the AC and PC components. The adherent mitral valve tissue appears thickened, myxomatous, and involved by blood cyst—the dark area of the PC. (An 8-week-old female infant with mild tetralogy of Fallot. Because of aortic overriding, fibrous LV outflow tract obstruction and fibrous subaortic stenosis were not synonymous, the outflow tract from the right ventricle to the aorta being widely patent. Reproduced with permission.[9]

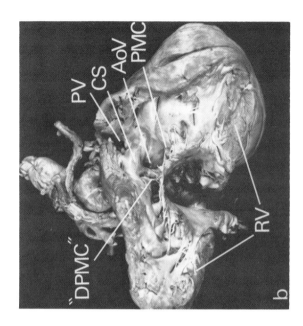

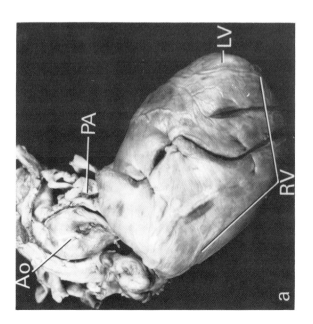

Figure 11. Tetralogy of Fallot with fibrous left ventricular outflow tract obstruction. **a**, exterior frontal view. Note the prominent right ventricle (RV), the relatively small pulmonary artery (PA), and large aorta (Ao), which are typical of tetralogy of Fallot. **b**, opened RV and PA. The conal septum or crista supraventricularis (CS) is displaced anterosuperiorly, with moderate narrowing of the outflow tract to the pulmonary valve (PV). The aortic valve (AoV) can be glimpsed beneath the anteriorly malaligned CS. The true papillary muscle of the conus (PMC) and a displaced or accessory PMC ("DPMC") are seen.

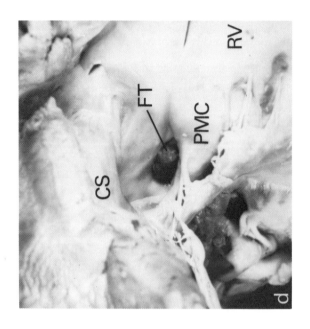

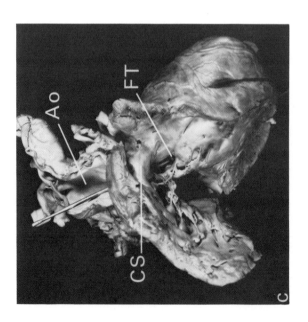

Figure 11c *shows a metal probe that has been passed from the left ventricle into the ascending Ao. In the expected site of the ventricular septal defect beneath the deviated CS, one sees instead a cuff of purple-black fibrous tissue (FT), surrounding the probe.* **d** *is a close-up of the dark-colored FT, above the PMC and below the CS, that occludes the ventricular septal defect to a major degree.*

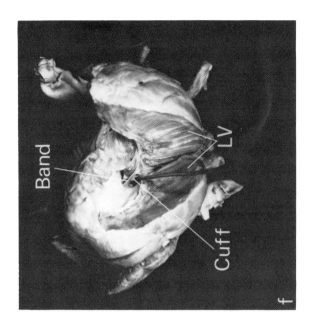

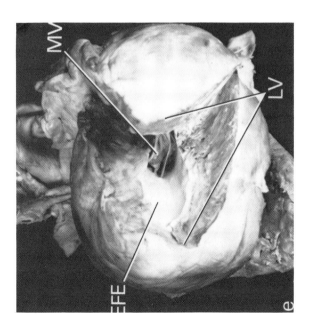

Figure 11e. *shows that the left ventricule (LV) is small-chambered and very thick-walled, with severe endocardial fibroelastosis (EFE). A fibrous band extends from the anterior leaflet of the mitral valve (MV) to the LV septal surface. f shows the cuff of fibrous tissue surrounding the probe in the LV outflow tract. (A 6-month-old white male infant; reproduced with permission.[9]*

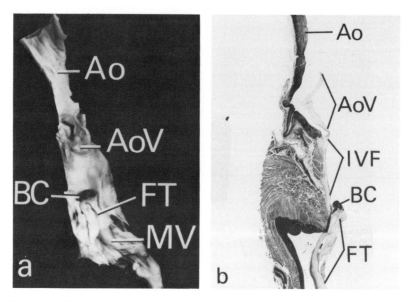

Figure 12. The fibrous left ventricular outflow tract obstruction seen in Figure 11 was excised for study. *a,* close-up photograph of excised specimen. *b,* photomicrograph of specimen, Verhoeff-Van Grieson stain, original magnification x 4.5. The obstruction was produced by a plug of fibrous tissue (FT), reminiscent of a bathtub stopper, that occluded the LV outflow tract and the ventricular septal defect from the left side. The plug looked black from the right ventricular side because it was surmounted by a purple-black blood cyst (BC). The FT was directly continuous with the anterior leaflet of the mitral valve (MV). Again, the fibrous tissue obstructing the LV outflow tract is intimately related to the MV; i.e., essentially excessive, redundant MV tissue. Ao, aorta; AoV, aortic valve; IVF, intervalvular fibrosa (between AoV and MV). (Reproduced with permission.[9])

over one year of age were from the computerized records of the Department of Cardiology of the Boston Children's Hospital. By 20 years of age onward, congenital AS was the second most common form of congenital heart disease among patients seen—ventricular septal defect being the most common. The overall frequency of congenital AS in these data is 833 of 16,170 (5.2%).

Thus, the pathology frequency of congenital AS (2.6% of all congenital heart disease) is an underestimate of the true situation that pertains in life. We think that the reason for this is that there are quite a few relatively mild cases of congenital aortic stenosis that do not die and undergo autopsy at a children's hospital. Also, it is our impression that the medical and surgical management of patients with congenital aortic stenosis is successfully prolonging life in many of these patients.

Concerning surgical aortic valvotomy, it is necessary for the surgeon to be able to see the aortic valve because it does not lie in the expected plane, i.e., at right angles to the long axis of the ascending aorta. Instead, the plane of the unicuspid aortic valve is almost parallel to the long axis of the ascending aorta (Fig. 1). The unicuspid aortic valve is like a tiny, thick, fibrous cuff that is suspended from only one point, the left coronary/noncoronary commissure. Consequently, the small aortic orifice faces mainly anteriorly (ventrally), instead of superiorly (cephalad). It is as though the aortic valve were a "coat" hung up on a single hook located posteriorly and to the left (the LC/NC commissure). Consequently, blind retrograde aortic valvotomy can miss the aortic valve altogether. The instrument may plunge into the ventricular septum in front of the semivertically oriented aortic valve, doing neither harm nor good, as in one of our cases, or the instrument can make a hole in the floor of the anteriorly located right coronary artery, leading to fatal intraoperative hemorrhage, as in another case. Thus, in view of the semivertical orientation of the unicuspid and unicommissural aortic valve, direct vision of the aortic valve would appear to be desirable in order to facilitate an effective valvotomy.

Regarding *acuspid aortic valvar stenosis*, the case presented heretofore (please see Findings) indicates that it rarely is possible for congenital aortic valvar stenosis to have no recognizable leaflets as such—just amorphous masses of fibrous tissue. We suspect that postnatal maturation of such potential leaflets may occur. Had this patient survived, recognizable aortic cusp(s) might have developed; however, this is speculation.

This case of acuspid (acommissural) congenital aortic stenosis also proves that congenital absence of all three aortic commissures does not necessarily result in aortic valvar atresia. We had thought that rudimentary development, or absence, of all three aortic commissures might be the developmental basis of aortic valvar atresia, due to lack of separation of aortic leaflet tissue, which in turn could result in fusion—or lack of separation—of all aortic leaflet tissue, leading to aortic valvar atresia. In other words, absence of one commissure leads to a bicuspid aortic valve, often with congenital aortic stenosis. Absence of two commissures leads to a unicuspid aortic valve, typically with severe congenital aortic stenosis. Hence, absence of all three aortic commissures may lead to aortic valvar atresia, the tissue of all three leaflets being in common, i.e., unseparated by commissure formation, thus resulting in aortic valvar atresia. However, this case illustrates that the aforementioned hypothesis concerning the morphogenesis of aortic atresia is not necessarily correct because, in this patient, marked underdevelopment of all three aortic commissures was not associated with aortic atresia. Despite this very rare case of acuspid congenital aortic stenosis, we hypothesize that congenital absence of all three aortic valvar commissures may be the embryonic pathogenesis in most cases of aortic valve atresia. Deficiency or other abnormality of truncal cushion tissue could explain the findings in our rare case of acuspid congenital aortic stenosis. Expressed somewhat differently, even though the aortic leaflet elements are not separated because of failure of commissure formation, the leaflet elements may not conglutinate if they are deficient in substance or if they are otherwise abnormal.

What is congenital fibrous subaortic stenosis? In this study, it was:

1. a discrete fibrous ring in five cases (Fig. 7), and
2. an obstructive anterior leaflet of the mitral valve in two cases (Fig. 8).

These may seem like two curious unrelated diseases, until one realizes that from the developmental standpoint, they are in fact very closely related. The discrete fibrous ring appears to be a sequela of endocardial cushion tissue that is intimately related to the formation of the anterior leaflet of the mitral valve and the septum of the atrioventricular (AV) canal (i.e., the AV septum). The discrete fibrous ring is composed of fibrous tissue that normally is "cleaned up" following formation of the anterior leaflet of the mitral valve, the AV septum, and the subaortic vestibule. If such endocardial cushion tissue is not "tidied up," it persists as subaortic fibrous tissue that typically reaches from the anterior leaflet of the mitral valve to the interventricular septum (Fig. 7). Hence, this fibrous tissue is intimately related, from the developmental standpoint, to the anterior leaflet of the mitral valve (Fig. 8). Hence, congenital subaortic fibrous stenosis, in a broad developmental sense, appears really to be abnormal mitral valve fibrous tissue (Figs. 10-12).[6,8]

The surgical risks inherent in the resection of subaortic fibrous stenosis become clearer when one realizes that the fibrous tissue to be resected is intimately related to the mitral valve:

1. laceration of the anterior leaflet of the mitral valve, in 3 of our five cases;
2. surgical production of a septal defect in one of our patients with an LV-to-RA (right atrial) communication; and
3. surgical heart block, one case.

In one of our patients, an 11.5-year-old girl with the postrubella syndrome, the bottom of the aortic leaflets displayed marked fibrous thickening at their junction with the aortic–mitral intervalvular fibrosa. This form of ''sub''-aortic stenosis involved the inferior extremity of the aortic valve leaflets and could not have been excised surgically, except by *aortic valve replacement*.

Both cases of congenital fibrous subaortic stenosis produced by anomalous development of the anterior mitral leaflet also could not be treated effectively surgically, except by combining *mitral valve replacement* with resection of the excessive subaortic fibrous tissue.

Ketamine medication, which induces both somnolence and systemic hypertension, merits consideration in order to avoid devastating hypotension with sedation during cardiac catheterization. This led to death in one of our patients with supravalvar aortic stenosis (see Findings).

Operative Notes: In order for surgical operative notes concerning patients with congenital aortic stenosis, particularly valvar aortic stenosis, to be comprehensible and useful for subsequent review, the pathological anatomy of the congenitally malformed aortic valve must be adequately described, including: (1) orifice size, (2) annular size, (3) leaflet thickness, and (4) the state of the commissures. For example, it is *not* satisfactory to state only that the aortic valve is bicuspid. This inadequate description begs three questions (Table II): Which aortic commissure is absent or rudimentary? Which is underdeveloped? Which is normally formed? The simple and practical method of designating the aortic commissures that is used in this chapter is recommended: RC/NC, RC/LC, and LC/NC (Table II).

Summary

Three main anatomic types of congenital aortic stenosis were found in a series of 64 autopsied cases: (1) valvar, 80%; (2) subvalvar, fibrous, 11%; and (3) supravalvar, 9%. Valvar congenital aortic stenosis was classified in terms of the number of functional leaflets, which was the same as the number of effective commissures: (1) tricuspid (tricommissural), 4%; (2) bicuspid (bicommissural), 27%; (3) unicuspid (unicommissural), 67%; and (4) acuspid (acommissural), 2%. When the stenotic aortic valve was bicuspid, the RC/NC commissure was absent in 79%, while the RC/LC commissure was absent in the remaining 21%. Bicuspid aortic valves, in addition to having one commissure absent (usually the RC/NC), also often had underdevelopment of the RC/LC commissure (in half of our cases). When the congenitally stenotic valve was unicuspid, the only commissure of normal height almost always was the LC/NC (in 94%).

Fibrous subaortic stenosis accounted for 11% of this series and appeared to result from the presence of residual AV canal fibrous tissue.

Supravalvar aortic stenosis (Williams' syndrome) was found in 9% and appeared to be a manifestation of a widespread arteriopathy.

There was a marked male preponderance in valvar congenital aortic stenosis (3.5:1) and subvalvar fibrous stenosis (2.5:1), but not in supravalvar aortic stenosis (1:1).

The median ages at death in the various anatomic types of congenital aortic stenosis were very different: bicuspid valvar, 10 months; unicuspid valvar, 7 days; subaortic fibrous, 13 years; supravalvar, 19 years.

Thus, congenital aortic stenosis appears to include at least three different diseases: (1) valvar congenital aortic stenosis; (2) subvalvar fibrous, which appears to be residual AV canal fibrous tissue; and (3) supravalvar, which is just one manifestation of a widespread arteriopathy.

This series contains several rare or unique cases, which to our knowledge have not been published previously: a newly recognized association of preductal coarctation of the aorta with severe valvar congenital aortic stenosis, severe valvar congenital pulmonary stenosis, and massive biventricular hypertrophy; a case with acuspid and acommissural congenital aortic stenosis; and a rare form of parachute mitral valve, i.e., absence of the posteromedial papillary muscle group with a divided AV canal (not a common AV canal).

The frequency of congenital aortic stenosis is higher than the autopsy data suggest. In 2,492 autopsied cases of congenital heart disease, the frequency of congenital aortic stenosis was 2.6%. However, among living patients, the frequency of congenital aortic stenosis was twice as high: 5.2% in 16,170 patients with congenital heart disease. From 15 years of age onwards, congenital aortic stenosis was the second most frequently diagnosed form of congenital heart disease (16%–17%), second only to ventricular septal defect.

A clear understanding of the pathological anatomy of the various anatomic types of congenital aortic stenosis is important not only for accurate diagnosis, but also for more effective medical (balloon dilatation) and surgical therapy. The therapy of congenital aortic stenosis remains an important and incompletely solved problem.

Acknowledgments: The authors thank Margaret W. Stevenson for typing and Terence Wrightson, Michael Mantone, Domenic Screnci, and Leslie Partridge for photography.

References

1. Van Praagh R, Baño-Rodrigo A, Smolinsky A, et al: Congenital aortic stenosis: anatomic findings in 64 postmortem cases. *Am J Cardiol* (submitted for publication)
2. David J, Castaneda AR, Van Praagh R: Potentially parachute mitral valve in common atrioventricular canal: pathologic anatomy and surgical importance. *J Thorac Cardiovasc Surg* 84:178–186, 1982.
3. Williams JCP, Barratt-Boyes BG, Lowe JB: Supravalvular aortic stenosis. *Circulation* 24:1311–1318, 1961.
4. Beuren AJ: Supravalvular aortic stenosis: a complex syndrome with and without mental retardation. *Birth Defects: Orig Artic Ser* 8:45–56, 1972
5. Lababidi Z, Wu J-R, Walls JT: Percutaneous balloon aortic valvuloplasty: results in 23 patients. *Am J Cardiol* 53:194–197, 1984.
6. Van Praagh R, Corwin RD, Dahlquist EH, et al: Tetralogy of Fallot with severe left ventricular outflow tract obstruction due to anomalous attachment of the mitral valve to the ventricular septum. *Am J Cardiol* 26:93–101, 1970.
7. Fyler DC, Buckley LP, Hellenbrand WE, et al: Report of the New England Regional Infant Cardiac Program. *Pediatrics* 65(suppl):377–461, 1980.
8. Sanders JH, Van Praagh R, Sade RM: Tetralogy of Fallot with discrete fibrous subaortic stenosis. *Chest* 69:543–544, 1976.

CHAPTER 3

The Pathophysiology of Left Ventricular Outflow Obstruction

Alan B. Lewis, M.D.

Left ventricular outflow obstruction may be produced by stenosis of the aortic valve, by fixed or dynamic subaortic stenosis, by narrowing of the supravalvar ascending aorta, or by classic coarctation of the aorta. For this discussion, the physiological disturbances created by valvar aortic stenosis in childhood will be emphasized and used as a general model for the other types of obstruction to left ventricular outflow.

The Aortic Valve Orifice

Valvar aortic stenosis is one of the more common congenital cardiac malformations, occurring in 3%–6% of patients. It usually results from underdevelopment of the valve commissure between the right and noncoronary leaflets, thereby producing a bicuspid valve. As with other types of fixed obstructions, the flow across the narrowed and often eccentric orifice is dependent upon the left ventricular systolic pressure generated proximal to the stenosis. However, the magnitude of the pressure drop alone is inadequate to assess the severity of obstruction because pressure is affected by variations in flow. The interrelationship between the anatomic and physiological determinants of severity (i.e., orifice size, flow, and pressure) are summarized by the Gorlin formula:

$$\text{Aortic Valve Area (AVA)} = \frac{\text{Flow (Q)}}{44.5\sqrt{\text{mean systolic pressure difference (MSP)}}}$$

43

Thus, the flow across a stenotic valve is related directly to both the size of the valve orifice and the square root of the mean pressure difference across the valve:

$$Q = AVA \times 44.5\sqrt{MSP}$$

Similarly, the pressure drop across the aortic valve during systole is a function of the square of the flow but is inversely related to the valve area:

$$MSP = \left(\frac{Q}{44.5 \times AVA}\right)^2$$

A doubling of flow will produce a fourfold increase in the pressure difference generated across the stenotic valve orifice.

In the normal child, both the aortic valve orifice and cardiac output increase in proportion to body growth, represented as the body surface area. From birth to adulthood there is approximately a sevenfold increase in each of these values. A neonate with a normal aortic valve area of 0.5 cm² (i.e., 2.0 cm²/m² of body surface area) would have no pressure difference across the valve during systole. However, if the valve area failed to grow normally but merely doubled in size by adulthood to 1.0 cm² (i.e., 0.6 cm²/m²), then a mean systolic pressure difference of approximately 40 mmHg would be required to maintain normal resting cardiac output (Fig. 1). However, with moderate exercise the mean pressure differential would increase to >100 mmHg. As the valve area decreases, the slope of the relationship between pressure and flow rises sharply. Valve orifices of 0.5–0.7cm²/m² are considered to be severely obstructed and warrant early intervention.

Diastolic reserve in the left ventricle may be compromised in the presence of severe outflow obstruction. The reduction in left ventricular compliance is secondary to both hypertrophy and interstitial fibrosis. If the resultant increase in end diastolic pressure were associated with a concomitant elevation in left atrial mean pressure, pulmonary edema would be a frequent occurrence. This is generally avoided in patients with aortic stenosis by a large but transient increase in the "a" wave following atrial contraction. Thus adequate left ventricular filling is maintained by the so-called "atrial kick" with only a minor increase in the left atrial mean pressure.

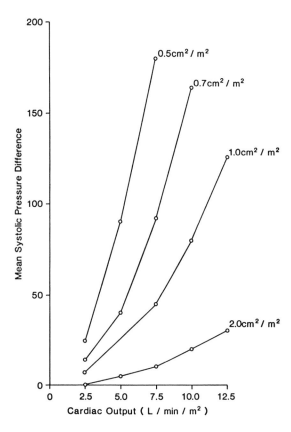

Figure 1. *The effect of increasing cardiac output upon the systolic pressure difference across a stenotic aortic valve is illustrated. As the valve orifice decreases, the aortic valve systolic gradient increases sharply in response to an exercise-induced elevation in cardiac output.*

However, such patients are particularly vulnerable to experience symptoms of congestive heart failure with the development of rhythm or conduction disturbances, which reduce or eliminate the contribution of atrial contraction.

Wall Stress and Hypertrophy

The elevation in left ventricular systolic pressure required to maintain normal flow in the presence of significant left ventricular outflow obstruction would result in a corresponding increase in wall tension were it not for the development of increased wall thickness.

The degree of left ventricular hypertrophy is related to wall stress by the Laplace equation:

$$S = P\frac{r}{h}$$

Wall stress(es) is proportional to both pressure and the left ventricular minor axis radius (r) but inversely proportional to wall thickness (h). Ventricular hypertrophy in most patients with valvar aortic stenosis is sufficient to normalize wall tension and compensate for the adverse effect of increased left ventricular systolic pressure. However, when hypertrophy is inadequate for the pressure load, wall tension, particularly peak systolic wall stress, rises. The adverse effect of elevated wall tension on myocardial oxygen requirements is reviewed in the following section.

Myocardial Blood Flow

Myocardial oxygen requirements rise in response to the increase in afterload generated by left ventricular outflow obstruction. The product of peak systolic pressure × heart rate can be determined readily in the clinical setting and has been shown to correlate closely with myocardial oxygen consumption. However, a better estimator of the oxygen requirements appears to be peak developed tension × heart rate. The area underneath the left ventricular pressure curve in systole also has been related to left ventricular oxygen needs and has been termed the systolic pressure time index (SPTI).

The subendocardial myocardium is particularly vulnerable to ischemic injury since maximal coronary vasodilation occurs earliest in this region. Further increases in subendocardial oxygen supply are limited by the relative lack of coronary vasomotor reserve as compared to the midmyocardium and subepicardium. Although it is possible that the early loss of autoregulation in the subendocardial coronary vessels is due to higher oxygen utilization, physical factors within the subendocardium appear to play a more important role. Intramyocardial compressive forces during systole have been shown to be greatest in the subendocardium, where they may equal or exceed intercavitary pressure and tend to decrease toward the epicardial surface. Thus, it is likely that there is little or no left ventricular subendocardial blood flow during systole,

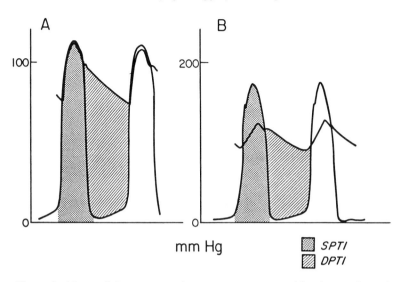

Figure 2. *Myocardial oxygen requirements are represented by the area beneath the left ventricular pressure curve during systole (SPTI) while oxygen supply are represented by the area between the aortic and left ventricular pressure tracings in diastole (DPTI). In aortic stenosis, SPTI increases but DPTI decreases.*

especially in the presence of aortic stenosis. Flow to the subendocardial muscle occurs, therefore, entirely during diastole. Once maximal vasodilation has occurred, flow to the subendocardium is dependent upon the coronary perfusion pressure and may be represented by the area between the aortic and left ventricular pressure curves during diastole (Fig. 2). This area has been termed the diastolic pressure time index (DPTI). This index of coronary blood supply can be converted into a measure of oxygen supply by multiplying DPTI by arterial oxygen content (DPTI $\times$ CaO_2). Left ventricular myocardial oxygen supply and demand may be estimated as:

$$\frac{DPTI \times CaO_2}{SPTI}.$$

A supply/demand ratio of approximately 20 is present in normal individuals. A critical reduction to 8 has been associated with

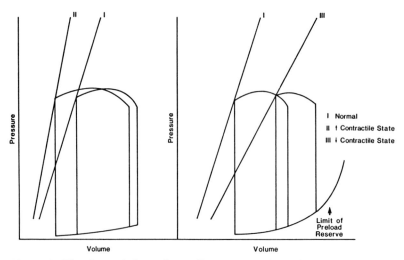

Figure 3. *The slope of the end systolic pressure-volume line is an index of ventricular contractility and is independent of loading conditions.*

inadequate subendocardial oxygen delivery. Reduction in this ratio may be produced by a decrease in coronary perfusion pressure (e.g., severe aortic insufficiency), anemia, hypoxemia or by an increase in left ventricular afterload, such as in aortic stenosis. It is important, however, that this concept of matching myocardial oxygen supply and demand not be oversimplified. Whereas a ratio of 8 appears to be a minimum limit below which subendocardial oxygenation will be compromised in normal hearts, this threshold may need to be increased in abnormal circumstances such as myocardial hypertrophy, ventricular dilatation, or inotropic stimulation. In the presence of severe valvar aortic stenosis and left ventricular hypertrophy, relief of outflow obstruction is essential, to maximize this ratio and insure the adequacy of subendocardial perfusion.

End Systolic Pressure-Volume Relation

The cardiac cycle of the contracting ventricle may be represented by a loop in which intracavitary pressure is related at any instant to ventricular volume (Fig. 3). An isolated ventricle beating isovolumetrically (i.e., at a constant volume) will generate a consistent

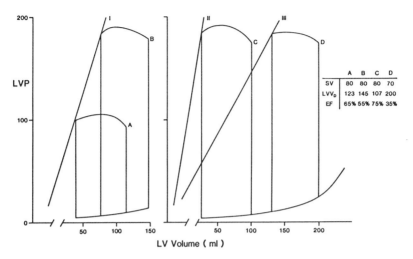

Figure 4. *Acute increases in LV systolic pressure will produce elevations in end systolic and diastolic volume (B). However, the gradual worsening of aortic valve stenosis can shift the end systolic pressure-volume line to the left (C). High LV systolic pressure then may be achieved without an increase in volume.*

pressure at end systole. Incrementally increasing the volume within the ventricle will produce a progressive linear increase in end systolic pressure. The slope of this pressure-volume line is an index of the contractile state of the ventricle and is largely independent of loading conditions, i.e., preload and afterload. If the ventricle is now permitted to beat normally, i.e., eject blood, it will reach the same point on the pressure-volume line at end systole. Increasing the contractile state of the ventricle will shift the slope upward and to the left, whereas a decrease in its contractility will be represented as a downward shift in the slope of the pressure-volume line.

Acute increases in left ventricular afterload result in an elevation in both end systolic and end diastolic volume in order to maintain stroke volume constant (Fig. 4). As we have seen from the Laplace relation, this causes a large increase in wall stress. However, the rate at which aortic stenosis worsens generally is slow, and compensatory hypertrophy is adequate both to normalize wall stress and steepen the slope of the pressure-volume line. This allows the left ventricle to achieve a higher systolic pressure despite a normal or even decreased end diastolic volume. Simultaneously, a normal stroke volume is maintained by a reduction in end systolic volume. Conversely,

Maturational Changes in Cardiovascular Function

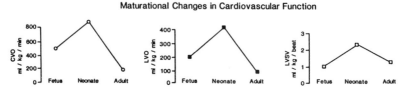

Figure 5. *The newborn experiences a doubling in LV output at birth. Flow/kg is even more impressive when compared to that of an adult.*

inadequate hypertrophy and/or reduced contractility result in a rightward shift in the slope. The Frank-Starling relation is used to maintain adequate cardiac output by increasing left ventricular end systolic and diastolic volumes. However, preload reserve is limited in severe aortic stenosis due to reduced compliance, and the ventricle quickly reaches the steep part of the diastolic pressure-volume curve. Further, small increases in end diastolic volume produce large increases in diastolic pressure. When diastolic reserve reaches its limit, maintenance of adequate systolic pressure may require an increase in end systolic volume. This is achieved, however, at the expense of reduced stroke volume. Thus, deterioration in left ventricular function in patients with severe aortic stenosis may produce the symptoms of clinical congestive heart failure, pulmonary edema, and low cardiac output. This is observed frequently in neonates with critical valvar aortic stenosis.

Aortic Stenosis in the Neonate

The neonate appears to have a limited ability to adapt adequately to the demands of severe valvar aortic stenosis. The normal newborn undergoes a profound increase in left ventricular output at birth (Fig. 5). Left ventricular output and stroke volume more than double when compared to the fetus. This acute change in the work of the left ventricle is even more impressive when the neonate is compared to an average adult. Thus, the normal newborn has considerably less functional reserve and is more likely to develop symptoms of congestive heart failure when faced with either pressure or volume overload (Fig. 6).

Newborns with critical valvar aortic stenosis may be divided into two categories based upon the size of the left ventricle (Table I).

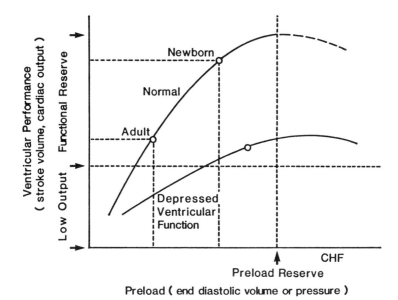

Figure 6. *The normal newborn myocardium functions at a significantly higher level than that of the adult and is close to the limit of functional reserve.*

Table I
Determinants Of Outcome in Neonates
With Critical Valvar Aortic Stenosis

Factor	Survival
LVEDV ≤60% PN	0
LVEDV >80%	85%
Dysplastic valve	33%
Aortic annulus 5 mm	0
LVEDV 140% PN	VF

Modified from: Edmunds, LH, Wagner, HR, Heymann, MA: Aortic valvulotomy in neonates. *Circulation* 61:421, 1980; Hammond, JR Jr, Parrish, MD, Graham, RP, et al: Risk factors for infants undergoing aortic vavotomy for critical aortic valvar stenosis. (Abstract) *JACC* 3:585, 1984.

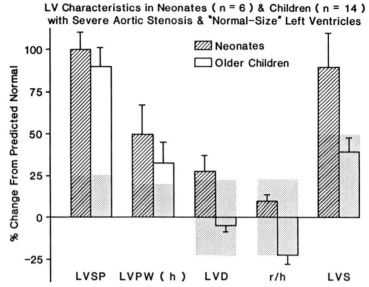

Figure 7. *Neonates with severe aortic stenosis and "normal-size" left ventricles have proportionately greater ventricular dimensions when compared to older children, which results in higher LV wall stress(es). The lightly stippled areas represent the normal range. LVSP = left ventricular systolic pressure; LVPW = left ventricular posterior wall; LVD = left ventricular minor axis dimension; r/h = minor axis radius/ wall thickness.*

Infants in whom the left ventricle is ≤ 60% of predicted normal have extremely low survival despite early valvotomy and probably represent part of the spectrum of hypoplastic left heart syndrome. When the left ventricle is more nearly normal in size (i.e., > 80% of predicted normal), survival is considerably improved. However, babies with dilated ventricles appear to be particularly susceptible to developing ventricular fibrillation. Review of the echocardiograms in a group of six newborns with critical valvar aortic stenosis and "normal size" left ventricles revealed proportionately less myocardial hypertrophy but more chamber dilatation when compared to older children. (Fig. 7). Estimated wall stress was approximately twice as high in the neonatal group and suggests that myocardial ischemia may be more significant in the very young patient.

Therapy

Medical management of the patient with severe aortic stenosis and congestive heart failure may be of limited benefit. Digitalis and other inotropic agents may improve left ventricular systolic function (i.e., shift the pressure-volume line upward and to the left), but they may also increase myocardial oxygen requirements and worsen the discrepancy between oxygen supply and demand. Similarly, diuretics may relieve the symptoms of pulmonary edema, but they also may reduce left ventricular preload in patients dependent upon the Starling mechanism and thereby decrease both stroke volume and cardiac output. Thus, if heart failure does not respond rapidly to the institution of medical therapy, immediate surgical intervention is essential.

Acknowledgment: The author gratefully acknowledges the secretarial assistance of Mrs. Nita Wiesenthal.

References

1. Edmunds LH, Wagner HR, Heymann MA: Aortic valvulotomy in neonates. *Circulation* 61:421–427, 1980.
2. Gaasch WH: Left ventricular radius to wall thickness ratio. *Am J Cardiol* f1 43:1189–1194, 1979.
3. Glanz S, Hellenbrand WE, Berman MA, et al: Echocardiographic assessment of the severity of aortic stenosis in children and adolescents. *Am J Cardiol* 38:620–625, 1978.
4. Hoffman JIE: Determinants and prediction of transmural myocardial perfusion. *Circulation* 58:381–391, 1978.
5. Lewis AB, Heymann MA, Stanger P, et al: Evaluation of subendocardial ischemia in valvar aortic stenosis in children. *Circulation* 49:978–984, 1974.
6. Rahimtoola SH: Valvular heart disease: the decision to treat. *Hosp Prac* 19:63–78, 1984.
7. Sagawa K: The ventricular pressure-volume diagram revisited. *Circulation Res* 43:677-687, 1978.
8. Spann JF, Bove AA, Natarajan G, et al: Ventricular performance, pump function and compensatory mechanisms in patients with aortic stenosis. *Circulation* 62:576–582, 1980.

CHAPTER 4

Congenital Aortic Stenosis: The CHLA Experience

Winfield J. Wells, M.D.

From 1962 to 1984, 114 patients underwent surgery for congenital aortic stenosis at Childrens Hospital of Los Angeles (CHLA). There were 73 males (64%) and 41 females (36%). For purposes of data presentation and analysis, the patients were divided into three subgroups according to their age at the time of initial operation. Seven patients (6%) were ≤ one month of age and comprised the *neonate* category. The *infant* subgroup included 15 patients (13%) and consisted of those who were > one-month and ≤ one-year old. The largest subdivision, classified as *children*, contained 92 patients (81%) who were between one and 17 years of age.

A majority of patients in each of the three groups presented with isolated valvar obstruction (Table I). Six (86%) of the seven neonates had isolated valvar lesions, while the seventh showed combined valvar and supravalvar obstruction. Similarly, with the exception of one with diffuse subvalvar stenosis, the remaining 14 infants (93%) exhibited isolated valvar lesions. While 56 (61%) patients classified as children demonstrated valvar lesions, obstruction was found at a variety of levels in the remaining 39 percent. Twenty-four children (26%) had isolated discrete subvalvar lesions, five (5%) had isolated supravalvar obstruction, and seven children (8%) had multiple level obstruction, which included three with combined valvar and subvalvar involvement, three with both valvar and supravalvar, and one occurrence of subvalvar and supravalvar obstruction.

Isolated valvar lesions were observed predominantly among males in the series. Isolated valvar stenosis occurred in 55 of 73 boys (75%) while seven boys (10%) had subvalvar, five (7%) had supravalvar, and six (8%) had combined lesions. Conversely, the females demonstrated a more equal ratio of valvar to subvalvar

55

Table I
Lesion type

	Neonate (N = 7)	Infant (N = 15)	Child (N = 92)
Valvar	6	14	56
Discrete Subvalvar (Membranous)			24
Diffuse Subvalvar (Hypertrophic)		1	
Supravalvar			5
Multiple Levels	1		7

Table II
Associated Cardiovascular Anomalies
(From Initial Cath Data or Autopsy)

Anomaly	No. Patients
Aortic insufficiency	31
Hypocontractile LV	16
Mitral insufficiency	8
Mitral stenosis	3
Pulmonary hypertension	7
Coarctation	6
Ventricular septal defect	7
Atrial septal defect	4
Patent ductus arteriosus	4
Miscellaneous	7
No associated anomalies	57

obstruction. Isolated valvar lesions were found in 21 girls (51%), and 18 (44%) had isolated subvalvar lesions. In fact, considering both isolated and combined forms, 20 females (49%) showed an element of subvalvar stenosis.

Cardiac catheterization or autopsy verified the existence of associated cardiovascular anomalies at the time of surgery in 57 patients (50%) (Table II). Four neonates (57%), eight infants (53%), and 45 children (49%) presented with associated disorders. Aortic insufficiency was the predominant lesion, occurring in 31 patients

Table III
Preoperative Symptoms

Symptom	Neonate (N = 7)	Infant (N = 15)	Child (N = 92)
CHF	7	10	7
Fatigue			24
Dyspnea			15
Angina			17
Syncope		2	9
Light headed			4
Arrhythmia		1	4
No symptoms		2	42

(54%). Hypocontractile left ventricle also was prevalent, being noted in 16 patients (28%). Five of these died, and subsequent autopsy proved endocardial fibroelastosis. Concomitant mitral valve disease, which proved to be a marker for poor outcome, was present in 11 patients, with insufficiency evident in eight cases and stenosis in three. Ventricular septal defect (VSD) was present in seven patients (12%), and aortic coarctation was present in six (11%). Atrial septal defect (ASD) and patent ductus arteriosus (PDA) were uncommon, each occurring in four cases (7%) in this series. Additionally, there were isolated occurrences of Marfan's syndrome, Wolff-Parkinson-White syndrome, and sinus of Valsalva fistula.

The younger patients in the neonate and infant categories were symptomatic in the preoperative period, while almost half of the patients over one year of age were asymptomatic. All seven neonates were in congestive heart failure as were nearly two-thirds (10/17) of the infants. Among children, 39 (42%) exhibited minor symptoms of fatigue or dyspnea on exertion, while only seven (8%) had consummate congestive heart failure. Forty-two children (46%) displayed no preoperative symptomatology. Noteworthy are the 18 children (20%) who experienced one or more anginal episodes, as well as the two infants and nine children in whom syncopal attacks were reported. Preoperative arrhythmia was uncommon, occurring in four children and one infant (Table III).

All operations in the series were performed using cardiopulmonary bypass. The gradient across the aortic outflow tract was measured preoperatively and intraoperatively after repair in 63 of the 114

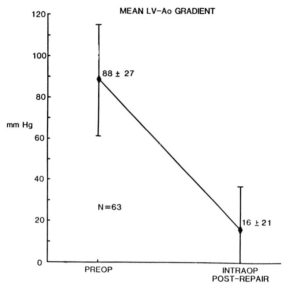

Figure 1. Mean left ventricular (LV) to aortic (Ao) gradient measured preoperatively at cardiac catheterization and postoperatively in the operating room following repair (Mean ± standard deviation).

patients. Preoperative gradients ranged from 40 to 160 mmHg, with a mean of 88 ± 27 mmHg. Intraoperative postrepair pressures ranged from 0 to 70 mmHg for a mean of 16 ± 21 mmHg. This mean pressure drop is depicted graphically in Figure 1.

Results

There were six hospital deaths (5%), five of the patients were four months old or less and the other was 20 months old. All those who succumbed had associated anomalies and were in severe congestive heart failure before operation. Two infants who died at surgery were in the first months of life and had concomitant mitral stenosis, pulmonary hypertension, and severe left ventricular dysfunction. One of these babies had subvalvar as well as valvar obstruction. Both deaths were attributed to low cardiac output, and at autopsy both were found to have severe endocardial fibroelastosis.

One infant and two neonates died perioperatively. Two had associated PDA and a small left ventricle as well as significant mitral insufficiency and pulmonary hypertension. In addition, one had an ASD while the other child had a coarctation. Both died of low cardiac output within two weeks of operation, which included ligation of PDA. The third patient who died perioperatively had valvar and supravalvar aortic stenosis and significant pulmonic stenosis. Following aortic and pulmonary commissurotomies and aortic patch angioplasty, the patient experienced a significant coagulopathy and eventually succumbed of low cardiac output.

The only hospital death in a child older than one year involved a 20-month-old who had a VSD and pulmonary hypertension in addition to valvar aortic stenosis. The VSD was not closed at the time of commissurotomy and the child died of arrhythmias and low cardiac output eight days after surgery.

Six patients (5%) were lost to follow-up from one month to eight years (mean, 3.8 years) after operation, for a comprehensive follow-up of 95% (108 patients). Excluding hospital deaths, 102 patients (89%) were followed from one month to 21.9 years through June of 1984, with a mean of approximately 10 years (122 ± 78 months).

Late death occurred in ten patients; a cumulative mortality of 15% (Table IV). All late deaths were in children more than one year of age at the time of their first surgery. The initial procedure in eight of the children was for correction of valvar lesions, one for isolated subvalvar lesions and one for combined sub- and supravalvar lesions. The interval to late death ranged from four months to 17.2 years after initial operation with a mean of 8.1 years.

Infection played a role in four of the ten late deaths. Two children had ruptured mycotic aneurysms; one of the aorta (expired four months postoperatively) and one of the brain (expired six years after aortic valve replacement and 17 years after initial commissurotomy). The third child had an intractable upper respiratory infection followed by cerebral infarct and brain abscess. Endocarditis destroyed the aortic valve 12.5 years postvalvotomy in the fourth patient.

Two patients died during a second reoperation (third procedure for aortic outflow obstruction). One child required an aortic prosthesis five years following initial commissurotomy. The artificial valve malfunctioned five years after implantation, necessitating surgery for replacement of the prosthesis, at which time he expired. The other child underwent a second commissurotomy 4.5 years following the

Table IV	
Late Deaths — Cause	
(N = 10)	
Infection	4
Residual AS* → Sudden death	2
Reoperation	2
Miscellaneous	2

*AS = Aortic stenosis

initial procedure and died five years later during attempted valve replacement for restenosis.

Sudden death was attributed to residual aortic stenosis in two cases. One patient died with a documented residual gradient of 50 mmHg, six months after initial commissurotomy. It was believed that further commissurotomy was not feasible. The second such death occurred 10 years postoperatively in a patient who had not received regular cardiac follow-up.

Another death occurred during childbirth 13 years postvalvotomy in a patient who had never been recatheterized. The final late death was attributed to arrhythmia eight months after aortic valve replacement, and seven years following initial aortic valvotomy.

Recurrent aortic outflow obstruction necessitated a second operative procedure eight months to 15.5 years (mean, 7.4 years) after the initial operation in one of five neonates (20%), four of 12 infants (33%), and 22 of 91 children (24%), for a total of 27 (25%) reoperated patients. Fifteen of the 27 (56%) had valve replacement and 12 (44%) had redo commissurotomies. The indication for reoperation was restenosis in 18 of the 27 (67%) and insufficiency in nine patients (33%). Of those who required a second procedure, the current status of 19 (70%) is very good, while six (22%) have undergone a second reoperation. Two late deaths (7%) include one patient who succumbed of arrhythmias six months after valve replacement and a second patient death that was not cardiac related.

When compared to patients with single level lesions, a greater percentage of patients who underwent primary surgery for the relief of stenosis at multiple levels required reoperation (Table V). Incidence of reoperation was 25% in patients who had isolated valvar stenosis, while 12% of those with only subvalvar stenosis and none of the five patients with isolated supravalvar obstruction have been reoperated. This is in marked contrast to the patients with obstruction at more

Table V
Reoperated Patients
(N = 27)

Lesion	Reop. Required
Valvar	19/76 (25%)
Subvalvar	3/25 (12%)
Supravalvar	0/5
Multi level	5/8 (63%)
3/3 Valvar & Subvalvar	
2/4 Valvar & Supravalvar	

than one level, where all three patients with combined valvar and subvalvar stenosis underwent reoperation (two commissurotomies for restenosis and one prosthesis for insufficiency), as did two of four patients with combined valvar and supravalvar stenosis (one redo commissurotomy and one prosthesis, both for restenosis). The interval to second surgery was significantly less in multiple level lesions where the mean was 3.4 years as compared to a mean interval of 7.4 years for all reoperations.

In our series, six patients (6%) have undergone a second reoperation (third surgery), at a mean interval of 4.5 years following their first reoperation and 9.5 years after the initial surgery. The indication for reoperation was prosthetic malfunction in two cases, insufficiency (requiring valve replacement) in one, and restenosis (two repeat commissurotomies, one valve replacement) in three. There were two hospital deaths, while the remaining four patients continue to do well two to 9.1 years (mean, 5.1 years) later.

One patient underwent three commissurotomies over approximately 11 years, and has required a third reoperation for aortic valve replacement secondary to insufficiency. Patient follow-up is summarized in Figure 2.

Survival curves have been constructed to access each of the three patient groups (Fig. 3). The incidence of hospital mortality was 29% (2/7) in neonates, 20% (3/15) in infants, and 1% (1/92) in children. As illustrated by the survival curve, actuarial probability of survival for neonates and infants is 71% ± 34% and 80% ± 20%, respectively, from the perioperative period through 15 years of follow-up. For children, the actuarial probability of survival up to 10 years after

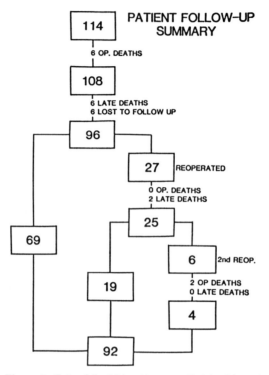

Figure 2. Fate of the 114 patients studied in this series.

surgery was 96% ± 4 percent. By 15 years, survival dropped to 86 ± 10%. The number of patients at risk has significantly decreased between 10 and 15 years, reducing the reliability of the data beyond the first decade of follow-up.

A curve depicting the probability of being "incident"-free has been constructed for each age group (Fig. 4). Infective endocarditis, reoperation, and death (hospital deaths included) were considered "incidents" in the construction of the graph. As is the case with the survival curve, the number of patients at risk in the neonate and infant categories severely limits the significance of their curves. The same holds true for the curve for children after approximately 13 years. Hospital death accounts for the initial drop in the neonate and infant curves. Neonates who survive surgery generally have done well through subsequent years while the infant curve suggests a progressive number of "incidents" scattered throughout the follow-

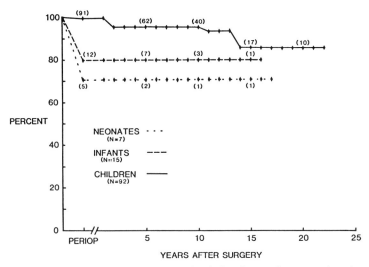

Figure 3. Actuarial curves for each of the three subgroups of patients based on age.

up period. Similarly, the curve for children reveals a gradual stepwise trend with an actuarial probability of being incident-free at five and ten years of 88% ± 8% and 71% ± 12%, respectively.

Iatrogenic aortic insufficiency is a major concern in the surgical correction of aortic stenosis, and we have tried to identify the incidence of surgically induced insufficiency in our series. Thirty-one patients (29%) had some degree of aortic insufficiency noted at initial evaluation. Twenty-three (74%) of that group had no postoperative increase in the severity of incompetence and have had no further surgery. The eight (26%) remaining patients have undergone reoperation; four (13%) for recurrent aortic stenosis (two redo commissurotomies and two prostheses), and four (13%) as a result of increased aortic insufficiency. The latter four patients required valve replacement from 2.7 to 14 years (mean, 8.4 ± 4.8 years) after their initial operation. Three are currently active and asymptomatic, while one patient died eight months following reoperation from arrhythmias associated with congestive heart failure (Fig. 5).

Thirty-one patients (29%) who had no mention of aortic insufficiency at initial evaluation were found to have some degree of

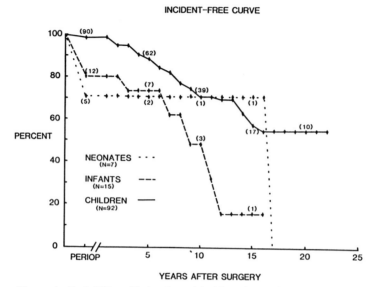

Figure 4. *Probability of being free of incident depicted graphically by the actuarial method ("incident" is defined as death, reoperation, or endocarditis).*

incompetence after their first surgery. In 27 (87%), the insufficiency was diagnosed as minimal, while in four it was felt to be significant. Of the 27 patients with mild postoperative aortic insufficiency (AI), two (7%) required reoperation for insufficiency. However, in both cases, bacterial endocarditis precipitated the progressive regurgitation, which ultimately resulted in prosthetic valve replacement. Of the four patients with significant postoperative AI, three (75%) have received prostheses as a result of aortic regurgitation at intervals of 10.7, 14.2, and 14.6 years following initial surgery (Fig. 6).

Although the incidence of bacterial endocarditis in patients with congenital aortic stenosis is low, the outcome has been poor in most cases. Six of our patients acquired endocarditis. One case occurred early after initial commissurotomy, and the patient expired four months later of a ruptured mycotic aortic aneurysm (previously mentioned). The five remaining cases occurred at a mean of 10.3 years after initial operation and resulted in one early endocarditis-related death and three subsequent aortic valve replacements for insufficiency (no AI prior to endocarditis).

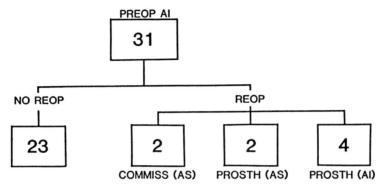

DIAGNOSED PREOP AI

Figure 5. Outcome in 31 patients who had aortic insufficiency noted at initial evaluation.

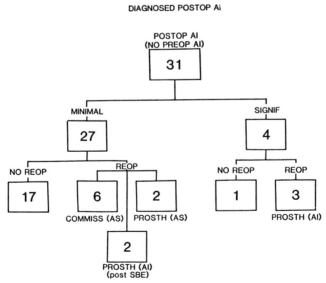

DIAGNOSED POSTOP AI

Figure 6. Outcome in 31 patients who had no aortic insufficiency noted at initial evaluation.

Conclusions

As a result of our review of patients with congenital aortic stenosis, the following conclusions have been drawn:

1. Surgery to relieve congenital aortic stenosis carries a low risk except in infants less than a few months of age, where hospital mortality approaches 25%.
2. Surgical mortality in congenital aortic stenosis is influenced not only by age, but by valve anatomy and associated cardiac defects such as concomitant mitral valve dysfunction.
3. There is a significant incidence of late death from cardiac causes following initial surgery for congenital aortic stenosis. Bacterial endocarditis has played a role in nearly half the cases of late death.
4. There is a decided incidence of reoperation after initial surgery for congenital aortic stenosis, with restenosis as the indication about twice as frequently as insufficiency.
5. Patients with obstruction at more than one level in the LV outflow tract require reoperation at a significantly higher rate than those with single level obstruction.
6. The mortality rate for reoperation is low, although a considerable number of patients require a third operation if the second procedure is a repeat commissurotomy.
7. Surgically induced aortic insufficiency is uncommon.

CHAPTER 5

The Use of Prosthetic Aortic Valves and Apical Aortic Conduits in Children

Gordon K. Danielson, M.D.

Although this chapter deals primarily with aortic prosthetic valves in children, data concerning other cardiac valves are included as well. The number of aortic valves replaced in children in any one institution is small; combining data from other valve positions increases the significance of the results and also allows some comparisons between valve positions. The discussion in this chapter will be limited to long-term results of prosthetic valve replacement in children.

Initially, we used the Starr-Edwards prostheses, almost all of the silastic poppet type. From May, 1963 to August, 1978, 50 patients 18 years of age or younger had received a Starr-Edwards prosthesis and had been discharged fom the hospital alive.[1] Nineteen patients had just aortic valve replacement, 24 received just a mitral prosthesis, and one patient had both. Six patients had tricuspid valve replacement; four of these had transposition of the great arteries, so that the tricuspid valve was the systemic atrioventricular valve. The ages ranged from six months to 18 years (mean = 10.4 years).

Twenty-four patients had undergone 29 previous operations (Table I). The majority of children undergoing valve replacement in the United States do not have rheumatic valve disease, in contrast to most other countries. In our series, many of the patients had valve defects as part of a complex congenital cardiac anomaly. The aortic valve dysfunction was principally insufficiency (19 of 20). In the mitral valve group, 20 patients had insufficiency, four had stenosis, and one had a mixed lesion. All six patients with tricuspid valve disease had valvular insufficiency.

Concomitant procedures performed in 22 patients are shown in

Table I
Prior Operations in Children Undergoing Starr-Edwards
Valve Replacement (24 Patients)

Operation	No. of Patients
Valvotomy or valvuloplasty	6
Repair of coarctation of aorta	6
Repair of tetralogy of Fallot	5
Repair of transposition of great arteries	4
Pulmonary artery banding	4
Repair of VSD and aortic insufficiency	2
Previous valve replacement	2
Total	29

VSD = ventricular septal defect.

Table II
Concomitant Procedures in Children Undergoing
Starr-Edwards Valve Replacement

Procedure	No. of Patients
Repair of truncus arteriosus	4
Graft replacement of ascending aorta	2
Patch enlargement of ascending aorta	2
Excision of subvalvular aortic stenosis	2
VSD closure	2
VSD closure, conduit repair of pulmonary atresia	2
Tricuspid valve anuloplasty	2
Repair of ostium primum ASD	1
Repair of complete atrioventricular canal	1
VSD closure, relief of pulmonary stenosis	1
Replacement of pulmonary artery homograft	1
Mitral valve anuloplasty	1
ASD closure	1

VSD = ventricular septal defect; ASD = atrial septal defect.

Table II. These included repair of truncus arteriosus, pulmonary atresia, and complete atrioventricular canal and conduit replacement of the aortic valve and ascending aorta. The sizes of the prostheses are shown in Table III. Many patients received an adult-sized aortic valve

Table III
Sizes of Prostheses in Children Undergoing Starr-Edwards
Valve Replacement

Size	Annulus diameter (mm)	No. of Patients
Aortic prosthesis		
7A	20	1
8A	21	1
9A	23	6
10A	24	4
11A	26	3
12A	27	2
13A	29	3
Atrioventricular prosthesis		
00M	20	4
0M	22	2
1M	26	2
2M	28	11
3M	30	8
4M	32	4

with or without aortic root reconstruction. Size 7A would be considered too small for adults; an 8A might serve for a small, relatively inactive adult. Approximately half of the atrioventricular prostheses would be considered adequate for adults.

The follow-up interval ranged from two to 17 years (mean = 7.9) and comprised 396 patient-years. Thirty-nine of 50 patients are still living; 30 are in New York Heart Association Class I, and eight are in Class II. Only one patient, in Class II, is unimproved. Late deaths occurred in three patients who had cardiomyopathy associated with atrioventricular valve insufficiency. The incompetent valves were replaced without affecting the cardiomyopathy, and all three patients died of progressive myocardial failure. Postmortem examination did not establish the cause of late, sudden death in two other patients whose cardiac prostheses were normal at autopsy. Complications of complex congenital heart disease caused late death in two patients.

Four patients were thought to have valve-related deaths from intracerebral hemorrhage, cerebral embolus, endocarditis, and valve dehiscence. The latter patient was in the early part of the series. The

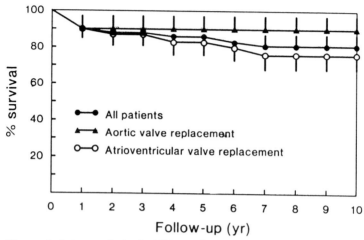

Figure 1. Late survival of children after Starr-Edwards replacement. Vertical lines indicate one standard error. (Reprinted with permission from HV Schaff et al.[1])

ten-year actuarial survival rate was 90% ± 7% after aortic valve replacement, and 76% ± 8% after systemic atrioventricular valve replacement (Fig. 1). These curves compare favorably with survival curves for our adult patients operated on during the same time interval.

Reoperation was required in four patients who outgrew their valves (all had atrioventricular valves). All survived reoperation, receiving an adult-sized prosthesis in all cases. None of the patients required reoperation for prosthetic valve dysfunction.

Nonfatal thromboemboli occurred in ten patients, half of whom were taking no anticoagulants at the time of their episode. Five had hemorrhagic problems related to anticoagulants, one serious enough to require hospital admission and blood transfusion. The overall incidence of late thromboembolism was 5.3 incidents per 100 patient-years after aortic valve replacement, and 2.0 per 100 patient-years after systemic atrioventricular valve replacement. The incidence of thromboembolism for aortic prostheses is similar to our own experience and that reported in the literature for adults operated on in the same era. In contrast, the thromboembolism rate for mitral prostheses in children was one-fourth that of our adult series, and one-half of the incidence for adults reported in the literature. Perhaps the relatively

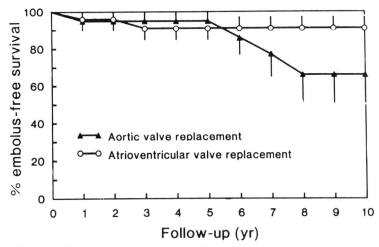

Figure 2. *Embolus-free survival after Starr-Edwards valve replacement in children. In the atrioventricular valve group, only patients with systemic atrioventricular valves were analyzed.* Vertical lines *represent one standard error. (Reprinted with permission from HV Schaff et al.[1])*

low incidence of atrial fibrillation in children accounts for some of the difference.

The embolus-free survival curves for Starr-Edwards prostheses in children are shown in Figure 2. It is interesting that the results after aortic valve replacement appear to be less favorable than those after mitral valve replacement. Perhaps a longer follow-up with larger numbers would eliminate this difference, as it is not seen in large series of adult patients.

As this series was being analyzed and the problems with thromboembolism and anticoagulants became more apparent, we switched to the Hancock glutaraldehyde-preserved porcine valve, which had just become available. From 1973 to 1980, 44 patients age 18 years or younger (range = 2–18 years, mean = 10.0) survived cardiac valve replacement with 46 Hancock valves.[2] The valves were placed in the following positions: mitral (16), pulmonary (10), aortic (8), tricuspid (6), left atrioventricular valve (2), and right atrioventricular valve (2). Two additional valves were inserted in the right atrial-inferior vena cava position in the early days of the Fontan procedure when such valves were thought necessary for a successful result. Concomitant procedures were performed in 32 patients (Table IV).

Table IV
Concomitant Procedures in Children Undergoing
Porcine Valve Replacement (32 Patients)

Procedure	No. of Patients
Ventricular septal defect repair	9
Right ventricular outflow patch	5
Atrial septal defect closure	5
Closure aorta-right atrial fistula	2
Right atrial-outlet chamber conduit	2
Ventricular septation	1
Atrial baffle	1
Other	7

The follow-up extended to 7.5 years (mean = 2.9) and comprised 113 patient-years. Thirty-seven of the 44 patients are living and well, but six of these required reoperation for valve replacement. One other patient died after reoperation elsewhere. The causes of the other six late deaths were: congestive heart failure, primarily related to the underlying complexity of heart disease (4), arrhythmia (1), and unknown (1).

Severe prosthetic valvular dysfunction necessitating valve replacement occurred in eight valves in seven patients, at 15 to 60 months postoperatively (mean = 34.1). This yields a calculated replacement rate for valvular failure of 7.1% per patient-year. The earliest failure necessitated an emergency reoperation for double valve replacement 15 months after the initial surgery. In addition to the seven patients who have undergone reoperation, there are presently six more who have newly discovered murmurs, indicating deteriorating valves. They undoubtedly will come to reoperation as well. We saw little difference in porcine valve deterioration between the left and right sides of the heart.

The one impressive advantage of the porcine valve is its remarkable freedom from thromboembolism; none of the patients in this series sustained this complication. In addition, patients are not at risk for anticoagulant-related bleeding. We believe that the complications of endocarditis and valve dehiscence are unrelated to the type of prosthesis used.

At the time tissue valves were introduced, it was not known that they would have an accelerated deterioration in children and that calcification could occur early, sometimes malignantly. In our series, the probability of a porcine valve remaining failure-free at five years is only 58% (Fig. 3). This experience with xenografts was sobering and led us to abandon the use of tissue valves in most children.

More recently, we have implanted the Bjork-Shiley valve in 33 patients with ages ranging from 6 months to 18 years. The mean follow-up is 41 months. Thus far, the results are about the same as one would expect with other prosthetic valves in the modern era. This valve does not seem to have clear advantages over the Starr-Edwards valve in terms of thromboembolism. There were also no mechanical failures in this group, but one patient required urgent reoperation for a thrombosed valve.

Encouraging progress in the prevention of thromboembolism in adult patients with mechanical valve prostheses recently has been achieved with antiplatelet agents. Dr. James Chesebro and colleagues reported on a prospective, double-blinded series, which was well controlled to be sure the patients were taking their medications.[3,4] They found there was a 1.2% incidence of thromboembolic events on warfarin alone, which this was reduced to 0.5% when dipyridamole (400mg/day) was added to the warfarin. The incidence of bleeding events essentially was unchanged (1.8% versus 1.6%). By contrast, addition of aspirin (500mg/day) to warfarin did not reduce thromboembolism (1.8%), but it significantly increased bleeding events (6.0%). Routine use of dipyridamole with warfarin in children has not been established, but antiplatelet therapy seems reasonable, especially for patients who have had suspected thromboembolism, particularly in the aortic valve group.

It is interesting that the incidence of thromboembolism in this recent series of patients on Coumadin alone is considerably less than for earlier series, a finding that other centers have also observed. It is clear that when comparisons are made between valves with regard to thromboembolic potential, the years of valve implantation and observation must be considered as well.

In summary, we have learned that in young patients with xenograft prostheses, there is a negligible incidence of thromboembolism without anticoagulants, but very poor valve durability. For this reason, the good long-term results with fresh homografts, as reported by Donald Ross and Brian Barratt-Boyes, have been of great interest. However, the lack of ready availability of fresh homografts in

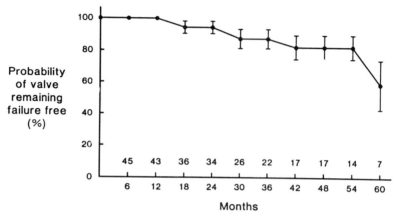

Figure 3. *Actuarial curve of probability of Hancock valve remaining free of the need for replacement, calculated according to the method of Kaplan and Meier. Numbers above the months shown on the* abscissa *are valves at risk. (Reprinted with permission from DB Williams et al.[2])*

most centers in this country has limited their use. Cryopreserved fresh homografts are now available, significantly improving the problem of availability. One hopes they will function as well as the fresh homografts, but it will be seven to ten years or more before we know how durable they are.

Mechanical valves function well in children, but we believe all patients should be carefully anticoagulated. The incidence of thromboembolism and bleeding in young patients is less than or equal to the incidence in adults, even though it may be more difficult to control anticoagulants in children. The tilting disc valve and the ball-and-cage valve both have excellent durability, and none in the above series have been replaced for mechanical failure. The addition of dipyridamole to warfarin decreases the incidence of thromboembolism. Dipyridamole and aspirin alone may provide an adequate, but probably less effective, substitute for warfarin if the latter cannot be used.

As for the use of left ventricle apical-aortic conduits in children, we believe it is unnecessary to perform this newer, more complex procedure on every patient with a narrow aortic root. There are a number of ways to enlarge the aortic root itself. We have had good results with a modified annulus-enlarging technique in which an oblique aortotomy is carried posteriorly and down through the noncoronary sinus to, but not into, the mitral annulus (Fig. 4). The incision is extended medially and laterally along the superior border of the annulus. It is not necessary nor desirable to incise the mitral valve. A generous patch can then be placed to enlarge the annulus at least 6 to 7 mm. We usually use pericardium for the patch. Recently, we have reviewed 100 patients who have had a pericardial repair to enlarge the aortic root.[5] None of the patches has become aneurysmal, and there have been no other late complications related to them.

We have seen several patients with prosthetic aortic stenosis after aortic valve replacement with small prostheses elsewhere. Shortly after operation, one such patient developed dark red urine as a result of severe hemolysis, and this was associated with anemia and angina. She was sent to us for consideration of an apical-aortic conduit. Her left ventricular outflow tract pathology was valvular-annular hypoplasia only, and by simply using this annulus-enlarging operation, we were able to remove the obstructive size 14 Lillehei-Kaster valve and replace it with a 25 mm Björk-Shiley valve. All her symptoms disappeared, and she is currently doing well. When dealing with valvular aortic stenosis, hypoplastic aortic annulus, prosthetic valve stenosis, and some cases of localized subaortic stenosis, the surgeon should keep in mind that root-enlarging procedures can often avoid a more complex operation.

In our series of 13 pediatric patients, we connected an apical-aortic conduit to the ascending aorta in seven and to the supraceliac abdominal aorta in six.[6] A diagram illustrating a left ventricle-to-abdominal aortic conduit is shown in Figure 5. The conduit passes through an opening in the diaphragm and then turns toward the midline to insert into the supraceliac aorta. The left ventriculogram shows the dye leaving the heart via both the ascending aorta and the conduit, meeting at the level of the aortic isthmus (Fig. 6). It was necessary to insert an apical-aortic conduit in only one adult patient in our experience. This man had severe calcified aortic stenosis and severe calcification of the ascending aorta, all the arch vessels, and the proximal descending aorta (porcelain aorta).

The 13 children had multiple diagnoses, including endocardial fibroelastosis (4), pulmonary stenosis (4), and ventricular septal defect (1). Twelve patients had one or more previous surgical procedures.

The left ventricular outflow tract gradient was eliminated in every case. The three infants who had associated endocardial

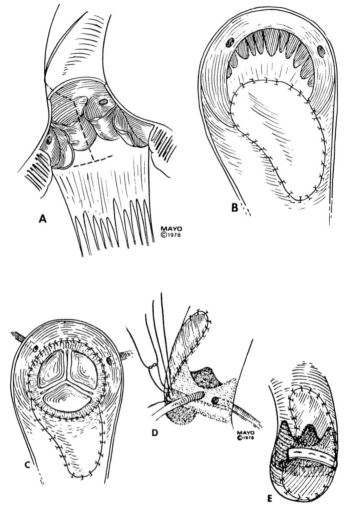

Figure 4. *Diagrams illustrating aortic root enlarging procedure.* **A.** *An oblique aortotomy is carried posteriorly down through the noncoronary sinus to the mitral annulus. The incision is extended medially and laterally along the superior border of the annulus* (anterior view).**B.** *A generous patch is sewn in place* (view from aortotomy). **C.** *The aortic prosthesis of choice is implanted* (view from aortotomy). **D.** *The valve may be tilted up posteriorly as shown to gain additional room for the sewing ring* (lateral view). **E.** *Valve sutures are passed from outside the aorta to the inside over a felt buttress in the area of the patch* (posterior view).

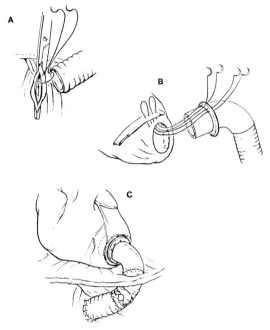

Figure 5. *Diagram illustrating a left ventricle apico-aortic conduit. A median sternotomy is performed and the incision is extended into the upper abdomen.* ***A.*** *A Dacron graft is anastomosed end-to-side to the supraceliac abdominal aorta over a side-biting clamp.* ***B.*** *Cardiopulmonary bypass is instituted and an opening is made at the left ventricular apex. A right-angle connector is sewn to the ventriculotomy over a strip of Teflon felt.* ***C.*** *The proximal conduit is anastomosed to the connector and led through an opening in the left hemidiaphragm. A distal conduit-to-graft anastomosis completes the reconstruction. (Reprinted with permission from RM DiDonato et al.[6])*

fibroelastosis and mitral insufficiency died (one survived two weeks but was ventilator-dependent). Such patients are currently not considered surgical candidates. Of the ten patients older than two years, there was one hospital death (10%). This patient had severe myocardial hypertrophy, and the heart could not be defibrillated after repair. This case illustrates the difficult problem of preserving the myocardium in patients with severe cardiac hypertrophy.

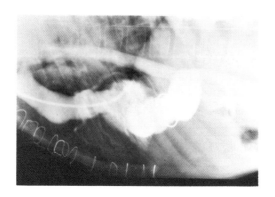

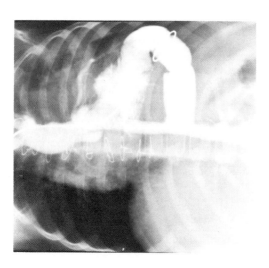

Figure 6. Left ventiriculogram after insertion of a left ventricle-supraceliac abdominal aortic conduit. *A.* Anteroposterior view. *B.* Lateral view. A thick, domed aortic valve is shown. There is no obstruction at the anastomoses or within the conduit. The stream of contrast material that passes through the native aortic valve meets the contrast material coming through the conduit and up the descending thoracic aorta at the level of the left subclavian artery. (Reprinted with permission from RM DiDonato et al.[6])

We used the Hancock porcine-valved Dacron prosthesis for the conduit in 13 patients. At last follow-up all but one of the survivors have required reoperation, usually from sudden conduit valve failure ("aortic" insufficiency). The interval to conduit failure was relatively short, ranging from 2.8 to 5.0 years, much shorter than for conduits on the right side of the heart in the right ventricle-to-pulmonary artery position. All patients had their porcine valves replaced with a tilting disc valve, and all are now on warfarin. Of great concern is the fact that, in some patients, the native aortic valve, which may have shown only minimal regurgitation initially, tends to develop progressive incompetence. One patient with an apical-aortic conduit required native aortic valve replacement, while the conduit valve remained functional. For these reasons, for patients who have tunnel subaortic stenosis and other unusual anatomical variations that cannot be handled by some type of aortic root reconstruction, we currently prefer the aortoventriculoplasty (Konno) procedure to the use of the tissue-valved apical-aortic conduit.

References

1. Schaff HV, Danielson GK, DiDonato RM, et al: Late results after Starr-Edwards valve replacement in children. *J Thorac Cardiovasc Surg* 88:583–589, 1984.
2. Williams DB, Danielson GK, McGoon DC, et al: Porcine heterograft valve replacement in children. *J Thorac Cardiovasc Surg* 84:446–450, 1982.
3. Chesebro JH, Fuster V, Pumphrey CW, et al: Combined warfarin-platelet inhibitor antithrombotic therapy in prosthetic heart valve replacement (abstract). *Circulation* 64(suppl 4):76, 1981.
4. Chesebro JH, Fuster V, Elveback LR, et al: Trial of combined warfarin plus dipyridamole or aspirin therapy in prosthetic heart valve replacement. Danger of aspirin compared with dipyridamole. *Am J Cardiol* 51:1537–1541, 1983.
5. Piehler JM, Danielson GK, Pluth JR, et al: Enlargement of the aortic root or anulus with autogenous pericardial patch during aortic valve replacement. *J Thorac Cardiovasc Surg* 86:350–358, 1983.
6. DiDonato RM, Danielson GK, McGoon DC, et al: Left ventricle-aortic conduits in pediatric patents. *J Thorac Cardiovasc Surg* 88:89–91, 1984.

CHAPTER 6

Update on the Technique of Enlarging Aortic Valve Annulus and Aortic Root

Albert D. Pacifico, M.D.

One of the more difficult problems that the surgeon must face is that of the hypoplastic aortic annulus and when to enlarge it. Since valve replacement must accompany annular augmentation, particularly when dealing with children, the surgeon must be concerned not only with early prosthetic hemodynamic performance but with the potential for late gradient problems associated with future growth of the patient.

It is certainly a serious iatrogenic problem to replace the valve of a child or an adult with an inadequate prosthetic device that leaves a significant gradient, thus creating an "aortic valve replacement mismatch." In Birmingham and in a number of selected centers around the world, when the aortic annulus size is 18 mm or larger, the cryopreserved or fresh aortic valve homograft can be inserted freehand without residual gradient.

In the past three years, our institution has been obtaining aortic valve homografts from patients with brain death, many of whom were serving as multiple organ donors.[1] The sterile cardiectomy is performed in the operating room, and the heart is transported at 4° C. Using sterile technique in an aseptic environment, the valve is removed from the heart along with the ascending aorta and the anterior mitral leaflet. To maintain leaflet viability the specimen is placed in modified Hank's solution, which contains physiological concentrations of antibiotics, for 48 hours. It is important not to use industrial doses of antibiotics because they alter the tensile strength of the leaflets, and the objective is to maintain leaflet viability. The valve is then stored by sealing it in a pouch with tissue culture media, initially subjected to controlled rate freezing to -40° C and subsequently stored indefinitely in liquid nitrogen at -196° C. The same basic technique is used by sperm banks. Studies performed in Brisbane, Australia, have demonstrated oxygen consumption of the leaflet tissue after defrosting valves stored for up to one year. Therefore, the technique may markedly improve valve durability when compared to homografts used earlier that were subjected to other methods of sterilization and preservation that destroyed the leaflet viability.

After defrosting the cryopreserved homograft in the operating room, the cylinder of aortic valve is tailored, excising the wall of the aorta in each of the sinuses. The remaining portion of the aortic wall is not viable and will calcify in time. The proximal edge of the valve beneath the leaflets is trimmed leaving a 2 mm cuff.

Our technique for homograft implantation begins with the placement of pilot sutures to orient the valve in the patient's aortic root. The homograft is rotated 120° so that the septal muscle portion of the annulus rests along the recipient left coronary sinus. The valve is then lowered into place, and each of the commissural posts are inverted into the ventricle, leaving the valve upside down and inside out. The proximal suture line is placed with a continuous technique at a level that corresponds to the nadir of each of the coronary sinuses and does not follow the normal scalloped annular configuration except in the area of the conduction tissue. The homograft commissural posts are then everted into the normal position and appropriately oriented relative to the coronary ostia. The distal suture line is placed with a continuous suture, as shown in Figure 1.

This operation can be done with a similar mortality rate as prosthetic valve replacement. The question that surrounds all the biological substitutes, however, is durability. The long-term results of this specific method of storage are unknown; however, using untreated fresh homografts, 90% of patients are free of cusp rupture at ten years.[2] We believe that this is probably the best substitute for isolated aortic valve replacement in a young patient whose aortic annulus size is 18 mm or greater.

The experience of Sir Brian Barratt-Boyes in Auckland, New Zealand, with 1,106 homograft valves placed between 1961 and 1981 showed a hospital mortality of 6.1%. This experience, dating back to 1961, includes an early period when myocardial protection was less optimal.

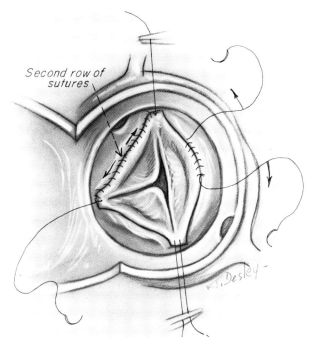

Figure 1. *The distal suture line of the homograft aortic valve is being completed. The valve has been rotated 120° counterclockwise. (Reproduced with permission from Kirklin and Barratt-Boyes.[3])*

Just as cardiac output is related to the gradient across a naturally stenotic aortic valve, so is it related to the prosthetic valve. Figure 2 shows the gradient in mmHg according to mean aortic valve flow in liters per minute for a standard Björk-Shiley valve of various sizes.[4] The 21 mm substitute has a significant gradient as the flow increases, although this is less so with larger size prosthetic valves.

A comparison of rest and exercise gradients across a 19 mm aortic prosthesis is shown in Table I. Note the left ventricular aortic gradient postoperatively. The various devices are listed, and the numbers in parentheses refer to the number of observations made regarding the specific substitute. We consider a gradient <10 mm at rest and <30 mm with exercise as a desirable performance of any prosthetic valve. The only device that has such low gradients is the Ionescu-Shiley

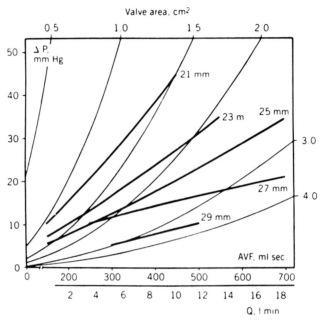

Figure 2. *Mean pressure differences across various sizes of Bjork-Shiley aortic prostheses and mean aortic valve flow (AVF) or cardiac output (Q). (Reproduced with permission from Bjork, et al.[4])*

pericardial valve, although the St. Jude valve approaches this. Because of premature degeneration, the heterograft devices are less suitable substitutes in children. If one must place a 19 mm device and a homograft is not available, the surgeon may opt to use the St. Jude valve or to enlarge the aortic annulus and place a larger sized substitute device. All of these data were compiled from adult patients.

Similar data are shown in Table II for 21 mm prosthetic valves. Again, only the St. Jude valve, the Hancock modified orifice valve, the Carpentier-Edwards valve, and the pericardial valve approach the desired postoperative hemodynamic performance. However, the heterografts and the pericardial substitutes, are not suitable for children because of premature degeneration.

If the root is less than 23 mm in diameter, it should be enlarged unless either a St. Jude or a pericardial bioprosthesis of 19 or 21 mm

Table I
Systolic Gradients Across Prosthetic Aortic Valves[+]

	LV Aortic Gradient*	
19 mm Device	Rest	Exercise
Björk-Shiley Standard	16 (24)	–
St. Jude	15 (9)	32 (6)
Hancock Heterograft	34 (8)	38 (7)
Hancock M.O. Heterograft	19 (6)	70 (1)
Ionescu-Shiley Pericardial	8 (3)	12 (3)
Desired Value	≤10	≤30

( ) = number of observations

* mmHg

[+] Modified from Kirklin JW and Barratt-Boyes BG: *Cardiac Surgery*. New York, John Wiley & Sons, 1986, p. 408.

Table II
Systolic Gradients Across Prosthetic Aortic Valves[+]

	LV Aortic Gradient*	
21 mm Device	Rest	Exercise
Björk-Shiley Standard	25 (33)	41 (20)
St. Jude	6 (5)	–
Hancock Heterograft	20 (18)	51 (12)
Hancock M.O. Heterograft	9 (46)	18 (7)
Carpentier-Edwards Heterograft	13 (5)	16 (1)
Ionescu-Shiley Pericardial	8 (6)	13 (6)
Desired Value	≤10	≤30

( ) = number of observations

* mmHg

[+] Modified from Kirklin JW and Barratt-Boyes BG: *Cardiac Surgery*. New York, John Wiley & Sons, 1986, p. 408.

is available and the patient is relatively small and inactive. In most adults, these devices will have significant gradients with exercise.

The surgical options available to manage the small aortic annulus are listed in Table III. The prosthesis may be inserted in the supra-annular position, which allows placement of a valve 2 mm in

---

Table III
Management of the Small Aortic Annulus

Surgical Options

Supraannular prosthesis
Supraannular enlargement by patching
Annular enlargement by patching
- Nicks
- Manouguian
- Konno-Rastan
Homograft replacement of the aortic root (Ross)
Left ventricular-aortic valved conduit

---

diameter greater than the actual annular measurement. The supraannular aorta may be enlarged with a patch, and then the prosthesis is tilted and placed so that it is sutured to the annulus in one part and then to the patch in the other part. This allows a 2–4 mm increase in size.

Methods of enlarging the aortic annulus began many years ago with a procedure described by Nicks[5] in which an incision was made through the noncoronary sinus and a patch placed across the aortic annulus, allowing enlargement of 2–4 mm in diameter. Another method of enlarging the aortic annulus posteriorly was described by Manouguian[6] and others. Still another procedure was described by Konno and Rastan,[7,8] where the aortic root was enlarged to the left of the right coronary artery and the interventricular septum also was enlarged by patching. A fourth procedure, replacement of the aortic root, was described by Donald Ross.[9] Finally, the aortic annulus can be bypassed with a left ventricular-to-aortic valve conduit.[10]

The operation described by Manouguian is shown in Figure 3. Looking at the aortic valve from the surgeon's view, the right and left coronary arteries and the anterior leaflet of the mitral valve are seen. An incision is made that passes through the commissure between the non- and left coronary sinuses. This incision, as originally described, can be extended into the anterior leaflet of the mitral valve, or it can stop in the area of fibrous continuity between the mitral and aortic annulus. In this figure the left atrium also has been opened. A patch is placed to enlarge the annulus, and a prosthetic valve is sutured into place. The left atriotomy is closed by suturing the left atrium to the

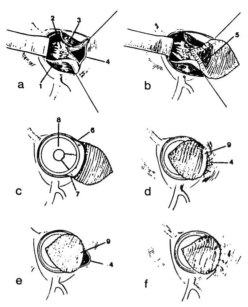

Figure 3. *Enlargement of the aortic annulus by posterior incision through the commissure between left and noncoronary sinuses (see text). (Reproduced with permission from Manouguian, et al.[6])*

patch. With this method, one can enlarge the aortic annulus in a simple way without increased surgical risk, and it accommodates a valve size between 4–6 mm, and possibly 8 mm larger than the actual annulus.

An autopsy specimen from a child is shown in Figure 4. The aortic annulus and valve are normal; the aorta is open. A posterior incision has been made between the left and noncoronary sinuses. The incision has been extended into the area of fibrous continuity but not through the hinged aspect of the anterior mitral valve leaflet. The circumference of the annulus has been enlarged about 15–16 mm, permitting insertion of a prosthesis of about 5 mm larger than the size of the native annulus.

Opening into the anterior mitral valve leaflet is probably contraindicated if there is mitral incompetence or a calcified mitral annulus. In addition, one must be concerned about an aberrant circumflex coronary artery, which may arise from the right coronary artery and course posteriorly, because it will be in the path of the

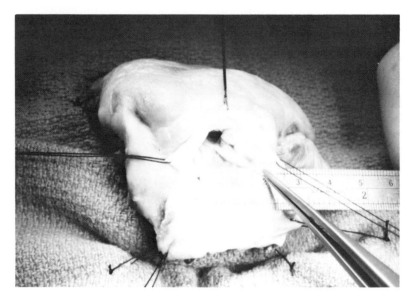

Figure 4. Autopsy specimen showing posterior enlargement of the aortic annulus (see text).

incision. If the mitral valve is widened, there will be some uncertainty regarding late postoperative mitral valve function.

Probably the most common technique used in children to enlarge the aortic annulus is the Konno procedure (Figs. 5,6). A longitudinal aortotomy is made that crosses through the annulus just to the left of the right coronary ostium, then extends into the anterior wall of the right ventricle and through the interventricular septum. A prosthetic aortic valve is secured posteriorly, and then a patch of Dacron is used to widen the incision in the septum and to form the anterior border of the prosthetic valve. The rest of the patch is used to widen the aortotomy incision. Finally, the right ventriculotomy is closed with a pericardial patch, which can be brought over the aortic patch to minimize bleeding. Dr. Ebert and his colleagues have published a series of 18 patients with one hospital death, a mortality of 6%.[11] One usually can place a 23–25 mm prosthetic valve, which should have a very low gradient even for an adult. The Konno operation has the advantage of maximally enlarging the annulus, while also relieving any subaortic component of obstruction.

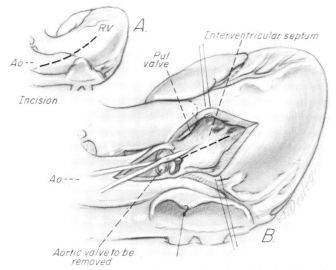

Figure 5. *Aortoventriculoplasty (see text for description). (Reproduced with permission from Kirklin and Barratt-Boyes.[3])*

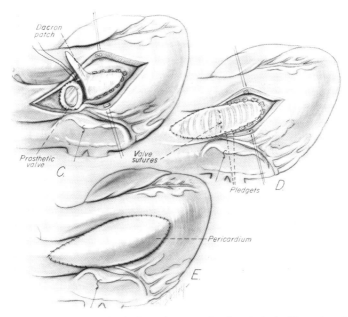

Figure 6. *Aortoventriculoplasty (see text for description). (Reproduced with permission from Kirklin and Barratt-Boyes.[3])*

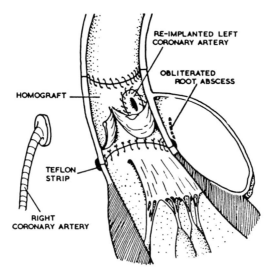

Figure 7. Homograft aortic root replacement with coronary artery reimplantation. (Reproduced with permission from Lau, et al.[9])

Potentially, injury to the conduction tissue or to the septal coronary artery may occur; however, left ventricular function is usually preserved.

Ross described a final method of enlarging the aortic annulus.[9] The aortic valve with the aortic annulus and a small portion of the ascending aorta is excised, and the ostia of the left and right coronary arteries are detached from the aorta. Then a cylinder of aortic valve homograft is sutured to the outlet of the left ventricle, beneath the aortic annulus, and the coronary arteries are reimplanted. The final result is shown in Figure 7. There is little worldwide experience with this particular operation, but it probably has some application.

We believe the use of a left ventricular-aortic extracardiac conduit should not be a primary surgical choice for this group of patients.

In summary, if one is planning to use a prosthetic device, we would recommend that a posterior annular enlargement be used when subaortic stenosis is absent and a suitable sized prosthesis can be placed by this method. When there is subaortic stenosis or a very small annulus, then the Konno operation should be performed.

References

1. Kirklin JK, Kirklin JW, Pacifico AD: Homograft replacement of the aortic valve. In: LW Stephenson (ed), *Cardiology Clinics*, Vol. 3, No. 3. Philadelphia, WB Saunders, 1985, pp 329–341.
2. Barratt-Boyes BG, Roche AHG, Whitlock RML: Six year review of the results of the free-hand aortic valve relacement using an antibiotic sterilized homograft valve. *Circualtion* 55:353, 1977.
3. Kirklin JW, Barratt-Boyes BG: *Cardiac Surgery*. New York, John Wiley & Sons, 1986, pp 373-429.
4. Bjork VO, Henze A, Holmgren A: Five years' experience with the Bjork-Shiley tilting-disc valve in isolated aortic valvular disease.*J Thorac Cardiovasc Surg* 68:393, 1974.
5. Nicks R, Cartmill T, Bernstein L: Hypoplasia of the aortic root. *Thorax* 25:339, 1970.
6. Manouguian S, Seybold-Epting W: Patch enlargement of the aortic valve ring by extending the aortic incision into the anterior mitral leaflet: new operative technique. *J Thorac Cardiovasc Surg* 78:402, 1979.
7. Konno S, Imai Y, Iida Y, et al: New method for prosthetic valve replacement in congenital aortic stenosis associated with hypoplasia of the aortic valve ring. *J Thorac Cardiovasc Surg* 70:909, 1975.
8. Rastan H, Abu-Aishah N, Rastan D, et al: Results of aortoventriculoplasty in 21 consecutive patients with left ventricular outflow tract obstruction. *J Thorac Cardiovasc Surg* 75:659, 1978.
9. Lau JKH, Robles A, Cherian A, et al: Surgical treatment of prosthetic endocarditis. Aortic root replacement using a homograft. *J Thorac Cardiovasc Surg* 87:712, 1984.
10. Cooley DA, Norman JC: Severe intravascular hemolysis after aortic valve replacement. *J Thorac Cardiovasc Surg* 74:322, 1977.
11. Misbach GA, Turley K, Ullyot DJ, et al: Left ventricular outflow enlargement using the Konno procedure. *J Thorac Cardiovasc Surg* 84:696, 1982.

CHAPTER 7

Surgical Perspectives for Aortic Atresia

Leonard L. Bailey, M.D.

Aortic valve disease, particularly in small infants and children, presents a formidable dilemma. Aortic valve atresia may be the worst cardiac defect that an infant can be born with. Many newborns with this anomaly are never diagnosed, and I presume the incidence is higher than reported. It has been suggested that cardiac replacement might offer a reasonable treatment, and I think many of us agree.

Aortic valve atresia represents about 7.5% of those children in the New England Registry, although this number may underestimate the number of children born with the anomaly. The defect is the cause of about 25% of all cardiac deaths in the first week of life.

Donald Doty,[1,2] in pioneering work, used conduit reconstruction, hoping to gain extension of life for some of these babies. Behrendt,[3] Levitsky,[4] and, in the last few years, Norwood and Lang[5,6] have amassed quite an experience with palliative procedures designed to extend the baby's lives for some as yet undetermined length of time. Dr. Norwood provided a ray of hope for these infants by reconstructing the aortic arch using the pulmonary artery segment, then placing a shunt from the systemic circulation to the pulmonary arteries. Generous atrioseptectomy also is included. Since the incidence of concomitant coarctation may be as high as 70%–80%, Norwood now carries his reconstruction on around to the descending aorta, an important feature for early survival. If these children can be kept alive beyond the first few weeks, the outlook for their future might be improved.

Behrendt's[3] operation provides the option to reconstruct the whole aortic arch and proximal descending aorta. The problem is the size of the aortopulmonary shunt, which is unpredictable. If it becomes smaller, an additional systemic-pulmonary shunt may be

---

Table I
Orthotopic Cardiac Xenotransplantation in Neonates
Clinical Trials—Loma Linda University

- Hypoplastic left heart syndrome uniformly lethal
- Virtual absence of newborn human donors
- Broad laboratory experience
- Extensive institutional and external review
- Extensive immunological research and screening
- Absent long-term data for staged palliation

---

required early. If it should become too large, pulmonary vascular changes may develop and preclude a second-stage Fontan procedure.

Secondary operations, which have been suggested, are also palliative. They employ the Fontan principle of atriopulmonary connection. These children have a single right ventricle and, in this group of patients, atriopulmonary connections are least likely to offer long-term benefit.

Lang and Norwood's last published report[6] should be considered critically. It includes 35 patients in his program of staged palliative procedures. Thirteen of the 35 patients left the hospital after the first stage operation. On restudy, only six became candidates for further palliation; four had the second stage procedure with two remaining survivors. Functional status and ultimate mortality of early survivors remain unknown.

In a combined series between Boston and Philadelphia, there were 130 patients. We anticipate that the steep falloff in actuarial survival will plateau at about 20%–30%, which may be the best one could hope for in most surgeons' hands in the short term.

For some years we have been studying the option of cardiac replacement (Table I). Our clinical trials on xenotransplantation are predicated on the following: (1) hypoplastic left heart disease is uniformly fatal, and (2) donors of infant human hearts are extremely rare. If babies with hypoplastic left heart are to be salvaged, it is essential to find a readily available cardiac substitute. Extensive immunoscreening is too time consuming for human allografting. Besides, it would be most unusual to have more than one donor choice. Currently, there is no standard brain death diagnosis code for newborns.

At Loma Linda during the last seven years we have done

extensive immunological research on many aspects of cardiac transplantation. We have performed about 150 orthotopic heart transplants in our laboratory in newborn goat recipients, using size-matched goats, lambs and some pig donors. Initially we wondered what would happen to newborn transplanted animals if they received no immunosuppression. As had been predicted in the literature, survival was possible both with allotransplantation (mean, 53 days) and xenografting (mean, six days).

For about three years we experimented with various protocols for selectively manipulating host immune systems or the graft to see if we could prolong survival. Until the advent of cyclosporine, we were unable to satisfy our expectations. But in 1982, using cyclosporine alone, we had newborn allografted animals that reached full maturity. The oldest, now three years old, has gone through a full pregnancy with a normal birth, and that baby was transplanted as well. The xenografted group also was improved with cyclosporine, resulting in a fourfold increase in survival in the unmatched lamb to goat pairs. One xenografted animal on cyclosporine alone survived to 72 days and died of causes unrelated to rejection. Addition of pulse-dose steroid among the xenografted animals resulted in host survival to nearly six months. Most of the deaths, however, have been from graft rejection. We have not had problems with infection or neoplasm. We probably have undersuppressed the animals. In all of our laboratory experience, the grafts have grown appropriately with the animals. Anastomoses have grown properly.

In attempting to choose an appropriate and available donor species for infants with aortic valve atresia, we considered those whose DNA resembles that of the human. Gorillas, chimpanzees, and orangutans were unavailable. Baboons became the species of choice partly because they procreate well in captivity. To begin, we did a number of isolated heart perfusion studies using baboon hearts and human blood, baboon hearts and baboon blood, and for a positive control, goat hearts and human blood. We found that baboon hearts, regardless of the perfusate, did well for 12 hours in isolated heart pefusion studies, whereas the goat hearts failed immediately with a hyperacute rejection phenomenon. The HLA system of tissue typing was tried in baboons, and we learned that baboons share similar reactions to humans. We believe significant homology exists between baboons and humans. In testing a large series of newborn human cord blood samples, we found an absence of preformed

---

Table II
Orthotopic Cardiac Xenotransplantation in Neonates
Clinical Trials—Loma Linda University

Recipient Screening and Selection

- Hypoplastic left heart syndrome
- Detailed inclusion and exclusion criteria
- Stable on PGE₁ infusion
- ABO and HLA typing
- Lymphocyte crossmatch
- Mixed lymphocyte culture

---

antibody against baboons—an encouraging and helpful sign. With additional studies, we learned that it is possible to look at the humoral side of the immune pattern in baboons, as well as the cellular side, identifying a "best" baboon donor for a specific recipient.

For choosing baboon donors, we perform an exhaustive screening process before the subject is entered into the donor panel. Panel baboons are infant, size-matched females. Baboons are quarantined for 30 days and undergo echocardiograms, chest x-rays, etc. When the complete series is checked and signed off, baboons are entered into the donor panel.

The Institutional Review Board approved protocol for clinical trials of xenotransplantation includes rather stringent inclusion and exclusion criteria for selecting recipients (Table II). Hypoplastic left heart disease or aortic atresia must be unequivocally confirmed, and the patients must stabilize on prostaglandin infusion. Serum crossmatch, tissue and ABO typing, and mixed lymphocyte cultures are compared against the panel of baboon donors. These tests take 4–5 days, so they must be started expeditiously. The transplantation consent form is one page long and has been reviewed extensively by our institutional boards and by a number of outside review committees.

The donor heart along with the arch and much of the descending aorta is obtained using inflow occlusion and cold cardioplegia. Donor lymph nodes, spleen, thymus, aorta, and blood also are obtained and frozen, so the baby can be tested against the donor in vitro. In that way, extensive immune testing can be done postoperatively in order to follow the rejection pattern. The graft cold ischemic time is about

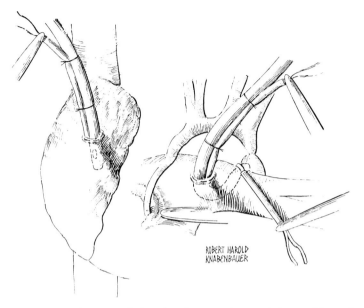

Figure 1. *Cardiac cannulation sites for operations on infants with aortic valve atresia. Whether for palliative reconstruction or for cardiac replacement, extracorporeal circulation is achieved by placing a venous cannula in the right atrium and an arterial cannula across the patent ductus arteriosus.*

two hours. The operation on the recipient baby is done with hypothermic circulatory arrest. The usual sternal-splitting incision is made, and the baby is perfused through the ductus to provide bidirectional flow in the aorta (Fig. 1). Although the left atrial cavity is small, the back of the left atrium has been quite adequate for atrial attachment. The recipient aorta must be widely opened past the ductus and well on to the descending portion to accommodate a long, bevelled strip of donor aorta, which augments the vessel and avoids any element of aortic obstruction. Pulmonary arteries are joined by simple end-end anastomosis (Fig. 2). The arterial perfusion cannula can be placed into one of the baboon arch vessels and the baby rewarmed. In our first human patient to receive a baboon graft, the heart started up intrinsically without defibrillation. Within a few minutes of rewarming it was maintaining excellent hemodynamics. Inotropic agents were not necessary.

Postoperative management in our first human baby included the

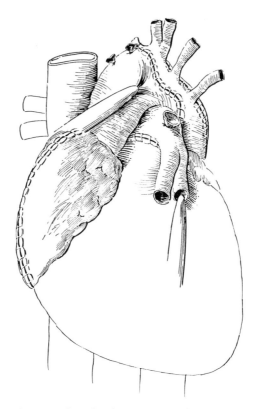

Figure 2. Completed appearance of orthotopically implanted cardiac graft. Note reconstruction of aortic arch beyond the patent ductus arteriosus using donor aorta.

use of cyclosporine with intermittent doses of steroid. Serial x-rays and ECGs were obtained along with daily echocardiography, which allowed a number of noninvasive indices to be followed. The battery of immune tests were important and interesting (Table III). We also obtained important information from enzyme testing. Our previous work with baboons had included CPK testing, and from this, a pre-MM fraction had been recognized as a significant marker. We followed this enzyme fraction in our clinical case and found it was a reliable indicator for graft injury.

Our first baby had a good initial recovery and lived 20 days. One mild and, perhaps, one moderate episode of "pre-rejection" were

---

Table III
Orthotopic Cardiac Xenotransplantation in Neonates
Clinical Trials—Loma Linda University

Laboratory and Immunological Monitoring

Lymphocyte sizing and differential
Helper/suppressor ratio
NK number and activity
Spontaneous blastogenesis
Mixed lymphocyte culture
Anti T and B Antibody
Immunoglobulin Level
Complement level

CPK Isozymes (especially pre-MM fraction)
Myoglobin Level

---

immunologically documented. These episodes seemed to do no harm to the graft. There was a remarkable lack of cellular infiltrate in the graft at autopsy. Rather, sheets of myocardial necrosis were apparent, which we have been unable to explain. We have been trying to duplicate in the laboratory what we found at autopsy, but so far we do not know why our patient died. Renal failure, which was present, remains a mystery since it should not have occurred with the doses of cyclosporine that were given. Infection was never a problem.

Review of the preliminary findings from autopsy showed that the heart was very compliant and not very enlarged. There was myocardial hemorrhage and cellular necrosis, but it wasn't the gritty, beefy heart of an ordinary transplant rejection. The atrial suture lines were clean on both sides, as were the aortic and pulmonary anastomoses. The left anterior descending coronary artery was slick and clean. Capillary sludging and areas of precapillary thrombosis were observed. There was no pulmonary edema, which correlated clinically with excellent blood gases within an hour of the patient's death.

The experience with our first clinical patient has led us to a careful evaluation of our efforts to this point. Based on this, we have decided to continue with our work, both in the laboratory and the clinical setting. What we have done is just another avenue of approach to this otherwise dreadful illness.

References

1. Doty DB, Knott HW: Hypoplastic left heart syndrome: experience with an operation to establish functionally normal circulation. *J Thorac Cardiovasc Surg* 74:624–630, 1977.
2. Doty DB, Marvin WJ Jr, Schieken RM, et al: Hypoplastic left heart syndrome: successful palliation with a new operation. *J Thorac Cardiovasc Surg* 80:148–152, 1980.
3. Behrendt DM, Rocchini A: An operation for the hypoplastic left heart syndrome: preliminary report. *Ann Thorac Surg* 32:284–288, 1981.
4. Levitsky S, van der Horst RL, Hastreiter AR, et al: Surgical palliation in aortic atresia. *J Thorac Cardiovasc Surg* 79:456–461, 1980.
5. Norwood WI, Lang P, Castaneda AR, et al: Experience with operations for hypoplastic left heart syndrome. *J Thorac Cardiovasc Surg* 82:511–519, 1981.
6. Lang P, Norwood WI: Hemodynamic assessment after palliative surgery for hypoplastic left heart syndrome. *Circulation* 68:104–108, 1983.

Editorial Comment

Masato Takahashi, M.D.

The problems of surgery for the unicuspid aortic valve. As noted in Dr. Richard Van Praagh's chapter, the number of patients with unicuspid aortic valves occupies a higher proportion than the actual occurrence reflecting the poor prognosis inherent in this subset of patients. Anatomically, not only does a single commissure lend support to the entire valve leaflet, the plane of the orifice tends to be parallel to the axis of the ascending aorta. When a surgeon attempts a "quick valvotomy" without adequate exposure, it is possible for him to miss the valve orifice entirely and intrude into the ventricular septum or the floor of the right coronary artery, leading to exsanguination. Even when the surgical instrument correctly engages in the valve orifice, a true commissurotomy is seldom possible; a tear may be produced anywhere along the leaflet.

Nevertheless, valvotomy without the use of cardiopulmonary bypass remains a preferred technique of some surgeons with a mortality rate of 20 percent to 30 percent. Despite the lack of true commissurotomy in such valves, many of the surviving patients appear to be effectively palliated.

The left ventricular-aortic conduit, as an alternative palliative treatment, may be considered as a temporary measure until a more definitive treatment can be used after the patient attains some growth. Problems inherent in such conduits include rapid calcification of the xenograft valve and kinking of the conduit brought about by growth of the heart.

Dilation of the unicommissural valve with the use of balloon valvuloplasty also is being tried. Thick valve tissue combined with unicommisural structure tends to make this subset of patients unpredictable. An extensive tear in the valve leaflet may cause significant aortic regurgitation. The margin of safety between success and failure in this form of treatment appears very thin, indeed. With further

101

clinical trials, this form of treatment may emerge as a viable alternative to surgery.

Enlargement of the aortic annulus.   In this chapter, Dr. Albert Pacifico discusses alternative ways to enlarge the aortic annulus. Basically, the choice is between the anterior and posterior approaches. According to Dr. Pacifico, if the patient clearly has a tunnel-type subaortic stenosis associated with a small aortic annulus, an anterior approach (Konno procedure) should be utilized and an appropriate vertical incision should be made. If no evidence of tunnel-type stenosis exists or if one is unsure whether the annulus should be opened anteriorly or posteriorly, then the aorta should be opened transversely.

Discrete subaortic stenosis.   Assessment of the subaortic region of the left ventricle under cardioplegia is not easy. Preoperative echocardiography is very useful in this regard. Careful assessment should be made with echo as to the nature of discrete subaortic stenosis and the degree of ventricular septal hypertrophy. During the operation, the fibrous ring may be removed as a block being careful to avoid damages to the mitral valve, ventricular septum, and the conduction system. Septal myomectomy or myotomy may be done as needed in the presence of ventricular septal hypertrophy.

Problems of cardiac transplant in newborns.   Cardiac transplant in newborns with hypoplastic left heart syndrome is receiving much attention. There are many problems facing surgeons attempting such a transplant. Limited availability of donor hearts is perhaps the severest constraint. However, there are plans to evaluate a small mechanical assist device that may put out a stroke volume as small as one cubic centimeter that will assist in the life support of recipient patients who are awaiting donor availability. Another serious problem is assessment of rejection. Currently, available biotomes are too large for babies weighing 2–3 kilograms. Myocardial biopsy in newborns is quite risky because of the relatively large size of currently available biotomes and the accuracy of noninvasive methods for detection of rejection has not been determined.

Section III
Transposition of the Great Arteries

There is fashion in operations as there is in sleeveless shirts.

George Bernard Shaw
The Doctor's Dilemma

Introduction

George G. Lindesmith, M.D.

Transposition of the great arteries is one of the more common congenital heart anomalies, but surgical therapy for this anomaly has been available only for a relatively short time. Consequently, there has been ongoing debate regarding the correct surgical approach to this anomaly. Initially, these discussions centered around various techniques for creating better mixing at the atrial level with surgery. With the advent of Rashkind's technique of balloon atrial septostomy, this concern diminished. Since that time, debate has centered mainly about the advisability of types of *atrial* switch operations and, more recently, the comparison with types of *arterial* switch operations.

This section begins with a scholarly presentation of the anatomic variations in transposition, followed by a chapter on the pathophysiology of the transposition complex. The remainder of the section is devoted to chapters regarding technique, mortality, morbidity, and short- and long-term results following the various available surgical procedures for treatment of transposition of the great arteries. Differing viewpoints are presented from both the cardiologic and the surgical points of view, and from these viewpoints one can derive that the final answer regarding the correct surgical approach to transposition of the great arteries is not yet available. These treatises, however, provide one with a well-rounded current view of the thinking regarding surgical treatment of transposition complex.

CHAPTER 8

Anatomic Variations in Transposition of the Great Arteries

Richard Van Praagh, M.D.

The anomaly now known as transposition of the great arteries was first described by Matthew Baillie[1] of London in 1797, and a second case was reported by Langstaff[2] in 1811. In describing the third known case in 1814, John Farre,[3] also of London, coined the term transposition of the great arteries (TGA). In 1875, Carl von Rokitansky[4] of Vienna reported corrected transposition. In 1898, Hermann Vierordt[5] of Tübingen described partial transposition, now known as double outlet right ventricle. TGA was then classified and reclassified by Abbott[6] (1915), Spitzer[7] (1923), Harris and Farber[8] (1939), and Cardell[9] (1956). In 1961 and 1962, Neufeld et al.[10–12] removed double outlet right ventricle from the category of TGA. In 1971, Van Praagh et al.[13,14] reintroduced Farre's[3] original meaning and definition of TGA, which has subsequently won general acceptance.

Definition:

Transposition of the great arteries (TGA) means that the aorta (Ao) originates from the morphologically right ventricle (RV) and that the pulmonary artery (PA) emerges from the morphologically left ventricle (LV). *Trans* is a Latin word meaning across, and *positio* is another Latin word meaning placement or position. Thus, "transposition" literally means "across placement." In TGA, both great arteries are "placed across" the ventricular septum and so rise above the wrong ventricles. In 1973, TGA was defined by Kirklin and his associates[15] as ventriculoarterial discordance. The terms and concepts of concordance and discordance had been introduced by Van Praagh et al.[16] in 1964.

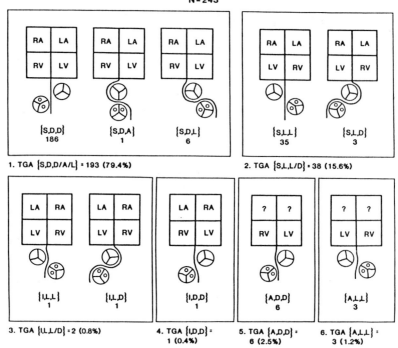

THE SIX MAIN ANATOMIC TYPES OF TGA
N = 243

Figure 1. The six main anatomic types of transposition of the great arteries (TGA): Diagrams viewed from above: ventral, toward bottom of page; dorsal, toward top of page; patient's right toward viewer's left hand; patient's left toward viewer's right hand; RA, morphologically right atrium; LA, morphologically left atrium; ?, morphologically unidentified atria; RV, morphologically right ventricle; LV, morphologically left ventricle; aortic valve indicated by coronary ostia; pulmonary valve indicated by absence of coronary ostia. Braces [ ] mean the set of.

[S,D,D] = the set of solitus atria (S), D-loop ventricles (D), and D-positioned great arteries. In D-loop ventricles, the RV is to the right (dextro or D) relative to the LV, and the pattern of anatomic organization of the ventricles is solitus (noninverted). In D-TGA, the transposed aortic valve is to the right (dextro or D) relative to the transposed pulmonary valve.

[S,D,A] = the set of solitus atria (S), D-loop ventricles (D), and A-positioned great arteries. In A-TGA, the transposed aortic valve is directly anterior (antero or A) relative to the transposed pulmonary valve.

[S,D,L] = the set of solitus atria (S), D-loop ventricles (D), and L-positioned great arteries (L). In L-TGA, the aortic valve (AoV) is to the left (levo or L) relative to the transposed pulmonary valve (PV).

TGA [S,D,D/A/L] = TGA with the set of solitus atria (S), D-loop ventricles (D), and D-positioned (D), or A-positioned (A), or L-positioned (L) great arteries. TGA [S,D,D/A/L] is physiologically uncorrected in view of the atrio-arterial alignments: RA with Ao (aorta), and LA with PA (pulmonary artery). In TGA [S,D,D/A/L], the atrioventricular (AV) alignments usually are concordant (RA to RV and LA to LV) and the ventriculoarterial (VA) alignments are discordant (RV to Ao and LV to PA) by definition, because TGA is present. Thus, in TGA [S,D,D/A/L], the segmental alignments typically are *solitus, concordant, discordant*. TGA [S,D,D/A/L] is by far the most common form of TGA.

[S,L,L] = the set of solitus atria (S), L-loop ventricles (L), and L-positioned great arteries. In L-loop ventricles, the RV is left-sided (levo or L) relative to the LV, and the pattern of anatomic organization of the ventricles is (or appears to be) inverted (i.e., a mirror-image of the normal or solitus pattern of anatomic organization). In L-TGA, the transposed AoV lies to the left (levo or L) relative to the transposed PV. L-TGA is (or appears to be) an inverted form (a mirror-image) of D-TGA.

[S,L,D] = the set of solitus atria (S), L-loop ventricles (L), and D-positioned great arteries (D).

TGA [S,L,L/D] = TGA with the set of solitus atria (S), L-loop ventricles (L), and L-positioned (L) or D-positioned (D) great arteries. No case of TGA [S,L,A]—solitus atria, L-loop ventricles, and A-TGA—was found in this series. In TGA [S,L,L/D], the TGA is physiologically corrected (associated malformations permitting) in view of the atrio-arterial alignments: RA with PA, and LA with Ao. The segmental alignments usually are solitus atria, discordant AV alignments, and discordant VA alignments; briefly—*solitus, discordant, discordant*. Thus TGA [S,L,L/D] is the classical form of physiologically corrected TGA and the second most common form of TGA.

[I,L,L] = the set of inverted atria (I), L-loop ventricles (L), and L-positioned great arteries (L).

[I,L,D] = the set of inverted atria (I), L-loop ventricles (L), and D-positioned great arteries (D).

TGA [I,L,L/D] = TGA with the set of inverted atria (I), L-loop ventricles (L), and L-positioned (L) or D-positioned (D) great arteries. TGA [I,L,L/D] is physiologically uncorrected TGA, as the atrio-arterial alignments indicate: RA to Ao and LA to PA. Segmental alignments typically are: inverted atria, concordant AV alignments, and discordant VA alignments, i.e., *inverted, corcordant, discordant*.

TGA [I,D,D] = TGA with the set of inverted atria (I), D-loop ventricles (D), and D-positioned great arteries. The segmental alignments typically are *inverted, discordant, discordant*; hence, TGA [I,D,D] is physiologically corrected TGA in situs inversus, in view of the atrio-arterial alignments: RA to PA and LA to Ao.

In segmental alignment analysis in TGA, one corcordant plus one discordant = physiologically uncorrected TGA; whereas two discordants = physiologically corrected TGA.

TGA [A,D,D] = TGA with the set of situs ambiguus (A) of the viscera and atria, D-loop ventricles (D), and D-TGA. In visceroatrial situs ambiguus, the state of the spleen must be stated, e.g,, asplenia, polysplenia, or normally formed.

TGA [A,L,L] = TGA with the set of visceroatrial situs ambiguus (A), L-loop ventricles (L), and L-positioned great arteries.

Segmental alignment analysis in TGA [A,D,D] and in TGA [A,L,L] is ambiguus atria, ambiguous AV alignments, and discordant VA alignments, i.e., *ambiguus, ambiguous, discordant*. (Ambiguus is the Latin adjective, modifying the noun situs. Ambiguous is the English adjective, modifying the noun alignments). (Based on Van Praagh et al.[17])

Findings

Main types. In 1977, in a series of 243 autopsied cases of TGA, six main anatomic types were found by Van Praagh et al.[17] in 1977 (Fig. 1).

1. *Physiologically uncorrected TGA in situs solitus* in 193 cases (79.4%), which consisted of TGA [S,D,D] in 186 cases, TGA [S,D,A] in one case, and TGA [S,D,L] in six cases;
2. *Physiologically corrected TGA in situs solitus* in 38 cases (15.6%), consisting of TGA [S,L,L] in 35 cases and TGA [S,L,D] in three cases;
3. *Physiologically uncorrected TGA in situs inversus* in two cases (0.8%), which consisted of TGA [I,L,L] in one case and TGA [I,L,D] in one case;
4. *Physiologically corrected TGA in situs inversus* in one case (0.4%), which was TGA [I,D,D];
5. *D-TGA in situs ambiguus,* which was TGA [A,D,D] in six cases (2.5%); and
6. *L-TGA in situs ambiguus,* which was TGA [A,L,L] in three cases (1.2%).

Infundibular (Conal) Anatomy in TGA

In 1980, Van Praagh et al.[18] found that in 221 autopsied cases of TGA of many different types, the conus was

1. subpulmonary in 0 cases;
2. subaortic in 212 cases (96%);
3. bilateral (subaortic and subpulmonary, with no semilunar-atrioventricular fibrous continuity) in seven cases (3%);
4. bilaterally deficient (deficient subaortic and subpulmonary conus, with aortic-tricuspid and pulmonary-mitral fibrous continuity) in two cases (1%).

Rarely, the infundibulum can be subpulmonary only—in TGA with posterior aorta.[13,14] Although present, the subpulmonary infundibulum in TGA with posterior aorta was very short.[13]

Thus, in strictly defined cases of TGA, it was found that the infundibulum almost always is subaortic only (96%), occasionally is bilateral (3%), rarely is bilaterally deficient (1%), and very rarely can be subpulmonary (in much less than 1% of cases). In our human data,[18] we found that the correlation coefficient (r) between TGA and a subaortic muscular conus (without subpulmonary muscular conus) equalled 0.83, the lower and upper 95 percent confidence limits being 0.79 and 0.86, respectively.

Subtypes

Associated anomalies can be of great importance in TGA. If one analyzes TGA not only segmentally, but also in terms of associated malformations, how many significantly different subtypes or subsets of TGA are there? In 1977, Van Praagh and his colleagues[17] performed segmental and associated malformations analysis in a series of 243 autopsied cases of TGA, the results are shown in Table I.

The frequencies of the six main types of TGA were (in order of decreasing frequency) (Table I):

1. physiologically uncorrected TGA in situs solitus, 79%;
2. physiologically corrected TGA in situs solitus, 16%;
3. D-TGA in situs ambiguus, 2%;
4. L-TGA in situs ambiguus, 1%;
5. physiologically uncorrected TGA in situs inversus, 0.8%;
6. physiologically corrected TGA in situs inversus, 0.4%.

The frequencies of the subtypes within the six main types of TGA were (Table I):

1. physiologically uncorrected TGA in situs solitus, 13 subtypes;
2. physiologically corrected TGA in situs solitus, 13 subtypes;
3. physiologically uncorrected TGA in situs inversus, 2 subtypes;
4. physiologically corrected TGA in situs inversus, 1 subtype;
5. D-TGA in situs ambiguus, 2 subtypes;
6. L-TGA in situs ambiguus, 2 subtypes.

Hence, in this series of 243 autopsied cases of TGA, six main types and 33 subtypes were found[6] (Table I).

Table I
Anatomic Types of TGA
N = 243

	Number	Percent
I. *Physiologically Uncorrected TGA in Situs Solitus*	193	79
1. TGA {S,D,D} with IVS	89	37
2. TGA {S,D,D} with IVS & PS	5	2
3. TGA {S,D,D} with VSD	38	16
4. TGA {S,D,D} with VSD & PS	16	7
5. TGA {S,D,A} with VSD & PS	1	0.4
6. TGA {S,D,D} with VSD & PA†	4	2
7. TGA {S,D,D} with VSD & preduct. coarc.	10	4
8. TGA {S,D,D} with TA†	6	2
9. TGA {S,D,D} with straddling TV	5	2
10. TGA {S,D,D} with single LV & DILV	6	2
11. TGA {S,D,D} with huge VSD (common V)	1	0.4
12. TGA {S,D,D} with MA†	6	2
13. TGA {S,D,L}	6	2
II. *Physiologically Corrected TGA in Situs Solitus*	38	16
1. TGA {S,L,L} with IVS	4	2
2. TGA {S,L,L} with VSD	3	1
3. TGA {S,L,L} with VSD & PS	2	1
4. TGA {S,L,L} with VSD & PA†	1	0.4
5. TGA {S,L,L} with AoA†, IVS, Ebstein's and Uhl's	1	0.4
6. TGA {S,L,L} With TA† (L)	3	1
7. TGA {S,L,L} with TS (L)	1	0.4
8. TGA {S,L,L} with straddling TV (L)	3	1
9. TGA {S,L,L} with single LV & DILV	12	5
10. TGA {S,L,L} with DIRV (L)	1	0.4
11. TGA {S,L,L} with MA† (R)	3	1
12. TGA {S,L,L} with MS (R)	1	0.4
13. TGA {S,L,D}	3	1
III. *Physiologically Uncorrected TGA in Situs Inversus*	2	0.8
1. TGA {I,L,L} with IVS	1	0.4
2. TGA {I,L,D}	1	0.4
IV. *Physiologically Corrected TGA in Situs Inversus*	1	0.4
1. TGA {I,D,D} with VSD & PA†	1	0.4
V. *D–TGA in Situs Ambiguus*	6	2
1. TGA {A,D,D} with asplenia	5	2
2. TGA {A,D,D} with polysplenia	1	0.4
VI. *L–TGA in Situs Ambiguus*	3	1
1. TGA {A,L,L} with asplenia	2	0.8
2. TGA {A,L,L} with polysplenia	1	0.4

Anomalies of the ventricles and of the AV valves were much more common with L-loops than with D-loops.

1. In TGA with D-loop ventricles, conotruncal anomalies only were found in 164 of 200 cases (82%). Additional anomalies of the AV valves were found in 36 of these 200 cases (18%).
2. In TGA with L-loop ventricles, conotruncal anomalies only were found in 11 of 43 cases (26%), whereas additional anomalies of the ventricular and AV valves were found in 32 of these 43 cases (74%).

Left ventricular outflow tract obstruction (LVOTO) was an important problem in TGA (Table I). In a previously unpublished study of 210 postmortem cases of TGA, we found the status of the LV outflow tract to be as follows:

1. no stenosis, 177 cases (84%);
2. LVOT stenosis, 30 cases (14%);
3. LVOT atresia, 3 cases (1%).

Of the 33 cases with LVOTO, the anatomic types of obstruction were

1. subpulmonary fibrous tissue, 15 cases (45%)
2. malalignment of the conal septum, 14 cases (42%);
3. both (1 & 2), 3 cases (9%);
4. acquired myocardial hypertrophy, 1 case (3%).

Conal septal malalignment producing subpulmonary and pulmonary annular stenosis is shown diagrammatically in Figure 2.

Ventricular septal defects in association with TGA can be

1. membranous, i.e., involving the membranous septum only;
2. conoventricular, i.e., between the conal and ventricular septa, with or without malalignment, with or without outflow tract obstruction (pulmonary or aortic), and with or without conal septal hypoplasia;
3. VSD of the AV canal type, with or without common AV canal, with or without straddling tricuspid valve, and with or without RV hypoplasia; and
4. muscular VSD, which can be single or multiple, small or

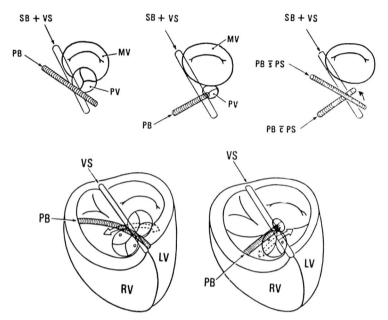

Figure 2. Conal septal malalignment. Comparison of the locations of the conal septum or parietal band (PB) in D-TGA with ventricular septal defect (VSD) but without pulmonary stenosis (PS) (left panel), and D-TGA with VSD with PS (right panel). When there is no PS, PB is located in the usual position, the posterior angle between PB and the plane of the ventricular septum (VS) and septal band (SB) being acute (30 degrees). Note that PB does not compress the pulmonary valve (PV) and subpulmonary outflow tract between itself anteriorly and the mitral valve (MV) posteriorly. Moreover, the VSD (indicated by the *arrow*) is subpulmonary. However, when PS is present (right panel), the entire conotruncus and the conal septum (PB) are rotated counterclockwise (as seen from above). Hence, PB runs much more posteriorly and leftward than usually, impinging upon the subpulmonary outflow tract and the pulmonary valve, and making the VSD subaortic (see *arrow*). The diagram in the upper right corner compares the locations of the "shifty crista" in the case without and with PS. (Reproduced with permission from Van Praagh et al.[17])

large, and can involve virtually any part of the muscular interventricular septum. Conoventricular VSD without malalignment is shown in Figure 3. Conoventricular VSD with malalignment is represented in Figure 4. VSD of the AV canal type and muscular VSD are shown in Figure 5.

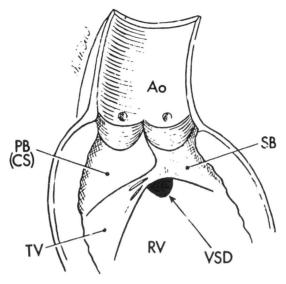

***Figure** 3.* Conoventricular VSD without conal *(infundibular) septal malaignment.* Right ventricular view showing the opened right ventricle (RV), aorta (Ao), the parietal band (PB) also known as the conal septum or crista supraventricularis (CS), and the anterior leaflet of the tricuspid valve (TV). This type of VSD lies between the conal septum, which is above, and the ventricular septum, which is below. It is often behind and slightly below the papillary muscle of the conus (to which TV is attached). When small, this type of defect is membranous and can be associated with an aneurysm of pars membranacea septi that bulges into the left ventricular outflow tract and can produce severe subpulmonary stenosis. This defect was found in 4.5 percent (5/112) of examined cases with VSD with the same frequency for D-loop and L-loop. (Reproduced with permission from Van Praagh et al.[17])

Discussion

1. *Data.* The large amount of data summarized here are of considerable clinical, pathological, physiological and surgical interest. They will not be reiterated. Suffice it to say that these data will repay careful study.

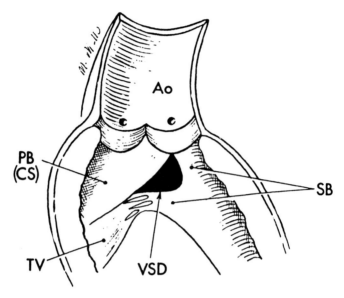

Figure 4. *Conoventricular VSD with posterior malalignment of the conal septum.* Opened right ventricle and aorta (Ao) showing the high subaortic VSD in the Y of the septal band (SB). The parietal band (PB) or conal septum (CS) is lying much more posteriorly than is usual. This leaves the space above SB wide open, resulting in a subaortic defect that may easily be mistaken for a conal septal defect. Typically, however, the conal septum is not deficient, but malposed—shifted abnormally leftward and posteriorly—too close to the mitral valve, thus crowding the left ventricular outflow tract and resulting in subpulmonary stenosis or atresia. This defect accounted for 27 percent (30/112) of examined cases with VSD. However, only 13 percent (4/38) of cases with VSD alone had this type; whereas 52 percent (11/21) with VSD and pulmonary outflow tract stenosis or atresia, and 70 percent (7/10) with VSD and preductal coarctation of the aorta had conal septal malalignment VSDs. (Reproduced with permission from Van Praagh et al.[17])

    2. *Method of data analysis.* Also noteworthy is the method of data analysis, which is based not only on the cardiac segments (Fig. 1), but also on the crucially important associated malformations.[19–22]

    3. *"Complete" TGA.* We prefer "physiologically uncorrected" TGA to "complete" TGA because, as has been understood since the

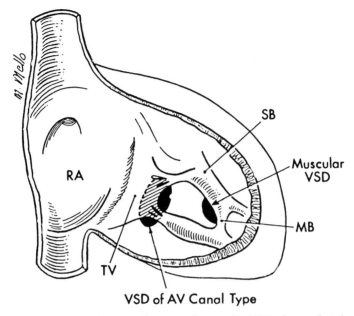

VSD of AV Canal Type

Figure 5. *VSD of AV canal type, and muscular VSD.* Opened right atrium (RA) and right ventricle showing muscular VSD in a characteristic site just inferior to the septal band (SB) and proximal to the moderator band (MB). This represents 5 percent (6/112) of examined cases with VSD. Also shown is a VSD of the AV canal type that is located medial to the "belly" of the septal leaflet of the tricuspid valve (TV). Of VSDs examined, 17 percent (19/112) were of the AV canal type. This comprised 30 percent (9/30) of the VSDs in TGA with L-loop and only 12 percent (10/82) in TGA with D-loop. AV = atrioventricular. (Reproduced with permission from Van Praagh et al.[17])

paper of Harris and Farber[8] in 1939, physiologically uncorrected TGA and physiologically corrected TGA both are complete TGAs. Physiologically uncorrected TGA typically is complete noninverted TGA, as in TGA [S,D,D] (Fig. 1). Physiologically corrected TGA typically is complete inverted TGA, as in TGA [S,L,L] (Fig. 1). All TGAs, as this term is now used, are complete. Partial TGA[5] is now called double outlet RV or double outlet LV. Since "partial" TGA has fallen into disuse, its opposite ("complete" TGA) is no longer necessary.

    4. *"Physiologically uncorrected" and "physiologically corrected" TGA.*

We think that these classical physiological designations are useful for the tabulation of large amounts of data, as in Table I. However, in our daily work, we do not use these old designations. We prefer diagnoses that are more specific and briefer, such as TGA [S,D,D] and TGA [S,L,L] (Fig. 1).

5. *Concordant or discordant*. We introduced the concordant or discordant concept in 1964,[16] and are in favor of it whenever it applies with accuracy. In all forms of physiologically uncorrected TGA, there is atrioventricular (AV) concordance and ventriculoarterial (VA) discordance (Fig. 1), at least in theory. Conversely, in all forms of physiologically corrected TGA, there is AV discordance and VA discordance (Fig. 1)—again, in theory.

The practical difficulty is that the *concordant or discordant alignment concept* often does not apply with accuracy because of the presence of associated malformations. Table I shows that the concordant/discordant concept did not apply in physiologically uncorrected TGA in situs solitus, i.e., in TGA [S,D,D/A/L], in 24/193 cases (12%), because of anomalies of the AV valves and ventricles. In physiologically corrected TGA in situs solitus, the concordant/discordant concept did not apply in 22/38 cases (58%). In TGA in situs ambiguus, the concordant/discordant concept did not apply in 9/9 cases (100%), because of the presence of situs ambiguus. For the series as a whole, the concordant or discordant concept did not apply in 55 of 243 cases (23%).

This series of cases (Table I) serves to exemplify why we have never proposed our concordant/discordant concept[16] for the classification of congenital heart disease as a whole, because there are so many anomalies to which the concordant/discordant concept does not apply. However, when accurate, we think this concept is satisfactory.

6. *Ventricular noninversion or inversion*. Initially, we wanted to use the noninversion or inversion concept to describe the anatomy of the ventricles, until we discovered that this concept has confused usage and can be meaningless. For example, it is generally agreed that physiologically corrected TGA has ventricular inversion. In visceroatrial situs solitus, this is clear: in TGA [S,L,L], it is generally agreed that the ventricles appear to be inverted (Fig. 1). In corrected transposition in situs inversus, i.e., TGA [I,D,D] (Fig. 1), the situation is far less clear: (1) One may view such ventricles as inverted for situs inversus, this is the visceroatrial-situs-dependent view or (2) one may

view these ventricles as noninverted in situs inversus; this is the visceroatrial-situs-independent view. Either way, the AV alignments are discordant. This is *why* we introduced the concept of AV concordance or discordance:[16] in corrected TGA in situs inversus, whether one prefers to view these ventricles as inverted for situs inversus or as noninverted in situs inversus, everyone could nonetheless agree that AV discordance is present. Then there is the additional problem of situs ambiguus. If one prefers the conventional visceroatrial-situs-dependent approach to ventricular diagnosis, then the concept of ventricular noninversion or inversion is meaningless when the visceroatrial situs (the frame of reference) is itself indeterminate.

Hence, using the conventional visceroatrial-situs-dependent approach to ventricular diagnosis, ventricular inversion means one thing in visceroatrial situs solitus (L-loop), the opposite thing in visceroatrial situs inversus (D-loop), and nothing in visceroatrial situs ambiguus. In the analysis of a large series of cases, as in Table I, it is essential that the meaning of diagnostic terms be clear, mutually exclusive, and unchanging. This also applies to computer programming: each term must mean one thing and one thing only, and meanings must never change. Otherwise, data analysis is impossible (or at least much more difficult and time-consuming).

7. *D and L terminology.* So this is why we introduced the D and L terminology to have simple, brief anatomic designations that are visceroatrial-situs-independent, always mean the same thing, and whose meanings do not change or become meaningless.

D-loop ventricles, L-loop ventricles, D-TGA and L-TGA, etc. (Fig. 1) have always been defined anatomically, and they were designed primarily for clinical diagnosis, as above.[19-25] These D and L designations also are meaningful embryologically, which is a considerable asset.[18,19,26,27] Clinico-pathologic-embryologic-etiologic correlation is one of the fundamental goals of research in congenital heart disease.

However, the greatest advantage of the segment-by-segment approach to diagnosis and designation in congenital heart disease is that this method always works easily and well. There are not a lot of anomalies to which it does not apply. The concordant/discordant approach to the diagnostic classification of congenital heart disease is a visceroatrial-situs-dependent approach, as are all the old diagnostic methods such as ventricular noninversion/inversion and physiologically uncorrected (noninverted)/physiologically corrected (inverted)

TGA. Being visceroatrial-situs-dependent, diagnostic meanings at the ventricular and great arterial levels therefore must change or become meaningless as the visceroatrial situs changes. The segmental approach to diagnosis is not just a different system of terminology. It is a new diagnostic method, one which is independent of changes in visceroatrial situs, which is why the segmental method of diagnosis always works. Each cardiac segment is diagnosed independently of all the others (Fig. 1). Then one mentally puts the segments together.

It is because of the use of this relatively new diagnostic approach—the segment-by-segment method and its visceroatrial-situs-independent D and L terminology—that the data in this series of 243 cases can be presented and analyzed so easily (Table I).

Some, however, prefer the AV and VA concordant or discordant approach.[15,28,29] For surgical purposes, when the congenital heart disease is not very complex, the concordant/discordant approach can work very well. When this sequential approach[28,29] breaks down, as in situs ambiguus and many other situations, its aficionados simply use the segmental approach.[19–22]

It should be added that the segmental approach[19–21] is sequential[28]: it proceeds in a logical venoarterial sequence from atria to ventricles to great arteries as in [S,D,D] (Fig. 1). The segmental approach to diagnosis, as in TGA [S,D,D], emphasizes the situs of the atria [S,-,-], the situs of the ventricles [-,D,-], and the situs of the great arteries [-,-,D]. It indicates the VA alignments specifically: TGA [-,-,-], but the AV alignments are implicit (unstated). When the atria are solitus and the ventricles are solitus or D-loop, one infers that the AV alignments are concordant: RA to RV and LA to LV (Fig. 1). If this is not the case, then the AV alignments are, of course, diagnosed specifically, as in TGA [S,D,D] with straddling tricuspid valve and VSD of the AV canal type.

In the sequential approach to diagnosis,[28,29] TGA [S,D,D] is expressed as solitus, concordant, discordant. The latter means that the atria are in situs solitus, the AV alignments are concordant (appropriate), and the VA alignments are discordant (inappropriate). The situs of the ventricles (D-loop) is inferred, and the situs of the great arteries is not stated or inferred.

The segmental approach,[19–21] as in TGA [S,D,D], emphasizes segmental *situs* analysis, whereas the sequential approach,[15,28,29] as in solitus, concordant, discordant, emphasizes segmental *alignment* analysis. Both segmental situs and alignment analyses are essential. Sequential analysis is a part of, and a modification of, segmental analysis. As indicated heretofore, there is no serious quarrel between these two somewhat different approaches. Although I am the blushing father of the concordant/discordant concept,[16] I prefer the segmental approach[19-21] to the sequential one, because the segmental approach always works, whereas the concordant/discordant approach does not—because the segmental method is visceroatrial situs independent, whereas the sequential approach is visceroatrial situs independent. The segmental approach does not break down, whereas the sequential approach does.

On the other side of the coin, some feel the sequential approach[15,28,29] is easier for beginners to master. This may be correct. However, our cardiologists, radiologists, surgeons, fellows, house staff and medical students have had no trouble learning the segmental approach that has been honed by daily use for two decades at the Boston Children's Hospital. I tend to think that physicians and surgeons can readily learn whatever it is that they are taught or decide to learn. I know from long experience that the segmental approach[19-21] (Fig. 1, Table 1) is easy to teach and easy to learn.

Finally, we are not talking about a contest between two rival diagnostic systems, with the reader as the judge. Segmental alignment analysis (the sequential approach) is just one part of the segmental method. The segmental approach is based on the (1) situs, (2) alignments, (3) connections, and (4) associated malformations of the cardiac segments,[19-22] as Figure 1 and Table 1 illustrate.

For those who do not like abbreviations, words of course, may be used instead. For example, TGA [S,D,D] means: transposition of the great arteries with the set of solitus atria, D-loop ventricles, and D-positioned great arteries. The segmental symbols are merely a convenience. Being Latin-based, this symbolic anatomy tends to transcend language barriers, whereas words may not.

8. *Alignments, not connections.* There has been a lot of imprecise talk about AV connections and VA connections, when it is AV alignments and VA alignments that are meant, accurately speaking. The atria do not connect with the ventricles, muscle to muscle, except at the bundle of His, because of the interposition of the fibrous AV canal or junction. The function of the fibrous AV junction is to connect and to separate, i.e., electrically to insulate the atria and the ventricles. The fact that the atria and the ventricles do not

connect directly is of great electrophysiological and developmental importance.

Similarly, the ventricles and the great arteries do not connect directly because of the interposition of the infundibulum or conus cordis. The fact that the ventricles do not connect directly with the great arteries is fundamental to the understanding of the conotruncal malformations. Maldevelopment of the conal connection appears to be the essence of the so-called conotruncal malformations.[18]

The atria, ventricles, and great arteries—the main cardiac segments (Fig. 1)—are like bricks, whereas the AV canal (or junction) and the infundibulum (or conus)—the connecting cardiac segments—are like mortar. The main cardiac segments (the bricks) do not connect directly. Instead, they are joined by the connecting cardiac segments (the mortar). Consequently, AV and VA alignments are preferred to AV and VA connections, when the meaning is what opens into what, in the interests of anatomic accuracy.

The main cardiac segments—the atria, ventricles, and great arteries (Fig. 1)—are *aligned* in various ways, whereas the connecting cardiac segments—the AV canal and the infundibulum—do indeed *connect*, accurately speaking. For example, in TGA [S,D,D] with straddling tricuspid valve (TV), the RA is *aligned* with both ventricles. But the RA does not connect with either ventricle because of the interposition of the fibrous AV junction. However, the straddling TV does connect the RA with both ventricles, muscle to muscle.

Hence, it is suggested that the concepts of segmental *alignments* and segmental *connections* be distinguished and used with anatomic accuracy.[21,22] This is highly relevant to the accurate diagnosis of TGA. In the classical form of physiologically corrected TGA (TGA [S,L,L], Fig. 1) for example, it has often been said erroneously that the AV *connections* are discordant. In fact, it is the AV *alignments* that are discordant: RA to LV and LA to RV (Fig. 1). It is noteworthy that completely discordant AV connections have never been described, i.e., tricuspid valve connecting only with the LV, and mitral valve connecting only with the RV, in the same heart. The concept of discordant AV connections is anatomically wrong. It is discordant AV alignments that is meant.

9. *TGA is a conal malformation.* The anatomy of the subarterial infundibulum was noted specifically in this presentation because TGA appears to result from maldevelopment of the conus cordis, not from maldevelopment of the aorticopulmonary septum as has long

been thought. The hypothesis that TGA results from conal maldevelopment was first proposed by Keith[30] in 1909, and was supported by ourselves subsequently.[18,31] The development of the aorticopulmonary (AP) septum is believed to be intrinsically normal in TGA. The AP septum is relatively straight, rather than spiral, in TGA, because the spatial relations between the great arteries proximally at the semilunar valves are very similar to the spatial relations between the great arteries distally at the level of the aortic arch/pulmonary bifurcation. Both proximally and distally, the aorta is anterior (ventral) and the pulmonary artery is posterior (dorsal); hence, the aorticopulmonary septum in typical TGA is relatively straight, rather than spiral.

The real question concerning the morphogenesis of TGA is not, "Why is the aorticopulmonary septum straight?" but rather, "Why is the aortic valve typically anterior (ventral) to the pulmonary valve?" Briefly, the answer, we believe, is abnormal development of the subarterial infundibulum, which typically is subaortic instead of being subpulmonary.[18,30,31] Development of the subaortic part of the infundibulum, instead of the subpulmonary part, elevates the aortic valve superiorly, protrudes it anteriorly above the RV, and widely separates the aortic valve from the mitral valve and LV. Lack of development of the subpulmonary part of the infundibulum typically results in the pulmonary valve being inferior and posterior, above the posterior LV, and in direct fibrous continuity with the mitral valve.

We have long known that straight development of the aorticopulmonary septum cannot possibly be the embryologic basis of TGA, despite the fact that the straight AP septum hypothesis is still the explanation found in almost all the books on congenital heart disease. What is wrong with the straight AP septum hypothesis? Well, it cannot account for the pathologic anatomic findings in typical TGA. It is true that one can "box the compass" with a malseptation hypothesis. Depending on how the AP septum grows downward, one can explain why the aortic valve is anterior to, beside, or posterior to the pulmonary valve—depending on the degree of twist of the AP septum.

However, the straight AP septum hypothesis cannot explain: (1) *the abnormality of the free walls of the great arteries*, as is indicated by the abnormal locations of *coronary ostia*, TGA being much more than an anomaly of the AP septum, because both the septum and the free walls are spatially very abnormal; and (2) *the variations in semilunar valve heights.* No AP malseptation hypothesis can explain why, with normally related great arteries, the pulmonary valve is high and the aortic valve is low; why, with TGA, the aortic valve is high and the pulmonary valve is low; why, with double outlet RV, both semilunar valves are high and approximately at the same height; and why, with double outlet LV, both valves are low and approximately the same height.

The malseptationists have attempted to explain these variations in semilunar valve heights by claiming that the subarterial infundibulum is part of the RV, and not part of the LV. The argument goes like this: of course, normal pulmonary valve and the transposed aortic valve are high, while the normal aortic valve and the transposed pulmonary valve are low, because the infundibulum is part of the RV and not part of the LV. Whichever great artery arises from the RV will have a high semilunar valve, and whichever great artery emerges from the LV will have a low semilunar valve.

What is wrong with that explanation? It is beautiful, except it is not true. The subarterial infundibulum (the parietal band or crista supraventricularis part) is not really part of the RV. The infundibulum (conus) is in fact a separate cardiac segment. It is true that the infundibulum normally becomes incorporated with the ventricles, mainly with the RV. However, one should not be misled by this. The infundibulum can straddle the ventricular septum to virtually any degree, because the infundibulum basically is not part of either ventricle. Although the infundibulum normally is incorporated mainly into the RV, it can straddle the ventricular septum to any degree (this anomaly is known as straddling conus), and the infundibulum can be located predominantly above the LV, as in anatomically corrected malposition of the great arteries,[32,33] and as in double outlet LV.[34] The ventricle that has the crista supraventricularis is not necessarily the RV (although it almost always is); the ventricle with the crista supraventricularis can be the LV.[32–34]

Thus, one cannot explain the semilunar valve heights in TGA by contending that the infundibulum is part of the RV and not part of the LV, because this contention is wrong, as the anomalies known as straddling conus, anatomically corrected malposition, and double-outlet LV indicate.

If TGA were due to a malformation of the AP septum only, and if the free walls of the transposed great arteries were normal, then the left coronary artery would be located normally (the coronaries being the first branches from the aortic free wall) and would arise posteriorly and to the left from the transposed pulmonary artery—which anatomically is not the case. In TGA, the coronary ostia typically are located normally relative to the aorticopulmonary septum, but the coronary ostia are very abnormally located in space relative to fixed external coordinates such as right-left and anterior-posterior, because the entirety of both great arteries (AP septum and aortic and pulmonary free walls) are very malpositioned. It has long been understood that transposition of the coronary ostia is an integral part of transposition of the great arteries.

Thus, although the classical straight AP septum hypothesis of the morphogenesis of TGA is initially appealing and seductive, it does not withstand close scrutiny (1) because it cannot explain the variations in semilunar valve heights; (2) because it cannot explain the abnormality of the great arterial free walls, as is dramatically demonstrated by the coronary ostia; and (3) because it cannot explain the one thing that all cases of TGA do have, namely, a malformed infundibulum. Finally, it is noteworthy that TGA virtually never has an aorticopulmonary septal defect (AP window). An AP window would be definite evidence that the AP septum *per se* is abnormal. We have never seen a case of TGA with an AP window.

For all of the foregoing reasons, we feel certain that in TGA, the AP septum is the sinned against, not the sinner—the victim, not the villain. Briefly, the straight AP septum of typical TGA is merely a secondary manifestation of the real problem, namely, that the aortic valve is anterior to the pulmonary valve because of malformation of the subarterial infundibulum.

10. *The infundibular malformation of TGA seems to have an important genetic component to its etiology.* We have been privileged to study the only good animal model of TGA that we are aware of, namely, the *iv/iv* mouse.[18,26,35] By "good" animal model we mean that not only is there a subaortic muscular infundibulum with aortic-atrioventricular fibrous discontinuity, but also absence of a subpulmonary muscular conus with pulmonary-mitral fibrous continuity. The *iv/iv* mouse (*iv* is the gene symbol for situs inversus) is a genetic model—thought to be a spontaneous mutant gene, maintained by inbreeding—not only of TGA, but also of double outlet right ventricle, common atrioventricular (AV) canal, polysplenia, and occasionally asplenia. The so-called *iv/iv* mouse model is now understood really to be an inbred genetic model of situs ambiguus, not of situs inversus. The

exact nature of the genetic abnormality in this model remains unknown.

11. *Set analysis.* There is a considerable difference among various segmental sets not only in terms of anatomy, physiology, and conduction system, but also in terms of associated malformations. For example, in TGA [S,L,L], of the 38 cases with discordant L-loops in situs solitus, 12 (32%) had single LV (absent RV) (Table I). By contrast, in the 193 concordant D-loops in situs solitus, single LV occurred in only 3%. Segmental set analysis, such as comparing TGAs with [S,L,L] segmental sets to those with [S,D,D] segmental sets, can be very illuminating. Why single LV is 10 times as common with TGA [S,L,L] as with TGA [S,D,D] is unknown at the present time.

12. *Classification of VSDs.* The classification of VSDs used in this study applies not only to TGA, but also to many different forms of congenital heart disease: (1) membranous, (2) conoventricular, (3) AV canal type, and (4) muscular (Figs. 3-5).

Future Directions

One may object that thus far I have stuck disgracefully close to my topic, that this chapter is overloaded with anatomic data. So now it is time to stick my neck out a little and *speculate* concerning where we are going in the future. We pay homage to data, but we really fly on intuition. When the big changes are made, there can be no data.

Which is better, the atrial switch or the arterial switch? Obviously I don't know the answer. No one knows at the present time, scientifically speaking. But what do I think? Briefly, I am very impressed with the arterial switch, because there are essentially no arrhythmias, as there most certainly are in the Mustard and the Senning. Perhaps the left ventricle and the mitral valve are better suited to support the systemic circulation for a lifetime than are the right ventricle and the tricuspid valve.

But one may object that for the first nine months of life prenatally, the right ventricle and the tricuspid valve handle systemic pressure and more flow work than do the left ventricle and the mitral valve. True, but prenatally the interventricular septum is approximately straight up and down (not markedly convex into the right ventricle or into the left) whereas, in TGA with intact ventricular septum, the RV becomes conical (as the LV normally is) and hence the ventricular septum bulges convexly into the low pressure LV. The tricuspid valve is able to occlude the right AV orifice prenatally when the ventricular septum is vertical.

But when the ventricular septum bulges away from the RV, creating a concave RV septal surface as the septum bulges convexly into the LV, then tricuspid regurgitation may well appear, because (we speculate) the tricuspid valve was never designed to occlude an approximately circular AV orifice, against systemic pressure, with a concave subjacent RV septal surface, armed only with relatively small papillary muscles.

Tricuspid regurgitation, for the aforementioned architectural reasons, may be as important as diminished right ventricular contractility as a cause of pump failure of the systemic RV in patients with TGA who have had an initially highly satisfactory Mustard or Senning procedure. At least, tricuspid (functionally "mitral") regurgitation, long-term, seems like one important concern regarding the atrial switch strategy.

Another is *diminished RV contractility*, independent of tricuspid function. You see, the RV contains a lot of functionally "dead wood," namely, the infundibulum. The contractile part of the RV is the true RV—the sinus, body, or inflow tract—not the infundibulum, conus, or outflow tract.

The *infundibulum* equals the parietal band (the distal or subsemilunar part of the infundibulum) plus the septal band (the proximal or apical part of the infundibulum). The distal or subsemilunar part of the infundibulum is the only part of the infundibulum that is involved in the morphogenesis of the conotruncal malformations, because this is the "switch" that normally crosses the circulations—or that fails to cross the circulations in TGA.[18] Hence, the subsemilunar part of the conus is there for developmental reasons, not primarily for physiologic reasons. This is also true of the septal and moderator band part of the RV apex. This is really the proximal or apical part of the conus, which is the "mother" of the RV developmentally. The RV sinus, body or inflow tract—the true contractile lung pump—evaginates out beneath the septal band.

The infundibulum (conus cordis or bulbus cordis) is the site of vertebrate adaptation to air breathing: (1) the crossing of the circulations by the distal conus (parietal band part) and (2) the development of a lung pump (the RV sinus) that pouches out beneath the proximal conus (septal band part).

Thus, much of the definitive RV—the proximal and distal infundibulum (septal and parietal bands, respectively) are there for structural and developmental reasons, not primarily for functional reasons. The infundibulum does contract, but not well. The infundibulum contracts with a "wringing action," as can be well seen in embryos. By contrast, the LV is all business, all function. It is the ancient professional pump. It really knows what it is doing. By comparison, the infundibular contraction is a late squeeze, not a swift kick. The foregoing observations are based in part on careful studies of chick embryos observed through dissecting and compound microscopes. I have made movies in time-lapse and real-time of the developing chick heart. The function, i.e., the relatively inefficient contraction, of the infundibulum has become apparent in relation to the Fontan procedure for tricuspid atresia and for single LV with an infundibular outlet chamber.

In assessing RV function, it is therefore important to distinguish between the true RV—the inflow tract proximal to the infundibular ring formed by the parietal, septal, and moderator bands—and the outflow tract (infundibulum), because the outflow tract normally is hypokinetic compared with a ventricle.

In TGA, the RV (inflow tract) often is relatively small. Most of the apparently good-sized RV is infundibulum. Functionally, this is not good news.

Below the AV valves, there normally are three chambers (not two): the LV, the RV (inflow tract), and the infundibulum (outflow tract).

Another potentially important consideration is that *the anatomic structure of the LV and RV free walls is very different*: the LV free wall consists of approximately two-thirds stratum compactum (coronary supplied myocardium) and one-third stratum spongiosum (trabeculae carneae); whereas the RV free wall architecture is the opposite: about one-third stratum compactum and two-thirds stratum spongiosum. The difference between the LV myocardial architecture and the RV myocardial architecture is understandable on a phylogenetic and ontogenetic basis (see Figures 3 and 4 of our single ventricle paper in 1964).[23] These well-documented structural differences between LV and RV myocardium strongly suggest that LV has more "bounce to the ounce."

Phylogenetically, this is hardly surprising. The LV is the ancient ventricle of the D-bulboventricular loop. All vertebrates have a ventricle, even ancient vertebrates such as the shark,[23] which is a cartilaginous fish (Chondrichthyes). Phylogenetically, sharks are much older than modern bony fish (Osteichthyes). By contrast, the RV is a specialization of the bulbus cordis. The RV appeared very much later in phylogeny, with the advent of air breathing.

Consequently, it would come as no surprise if it was to be proved physiologically that the RV is a less efficient pump than the LV. Indeed, it would be very surprising if this was not the case, in view of the fact that the true RV (the RV inflow tract) is smaller than the LV (which is almost all sinus), plus the fact that the infundibulum is hypokinetic (compared with the LV).

Then there is the problem of *functional left ventricular outflow tract obstruction* (LVOTO), with or without an organic component. Functionally, this resembles IHSS (idiopathic hypertrophic subaortic stenosis). The atrial switch strategy leaves the ventricular septum bulging convexly into the LV, predisposing to LVOTO, whereas the arterial switch cures functional LVOTO by restoring conical (as opposed to crescentic) LV architecture.

Thus, for many reasons, it appears desirable in the treatment of conotruncal malformations for the LV and mitral valve to support the systemic circulation. This does not have to be accomplished by great arterial and coronary translocation, as in the *Jatene procedure* for TGA.[36] *Intraventricular rerouting*, i.e., the *McGoon procedure*,[37] with or without infundibular septal resection, is another method of accomplishing the same end. Dacron conduits, with porcine homograft valves, appear to be very bad news long-term, because of the development of peel within the conduit, plus calcific degeneration of the porcine valve in the conduit. Arterial homografts may well prove to be much superior to Dacron conduits; however, more experience is needed.

Thus, as I peer into my imaginary crystal ball, it seems to me for many reasons that *appropriate ventricular repair of TGA* (and other conotruncal malformations)—resulting in a systemic LV and a pulmonary RV—either by means of arterial switching[38] or intraventricular rerouting, appears to have much to recommend it.

The main *dis*advantage of the arterial switch procedure appears to be coronary kinking. However, extensive dissection and liberation of the coronary arteries may well largely solve this problem of acute myocardial infarction intraoperatively and immediately postoperatively.

The advantages of the atrial switch procedures (Senning and Mustard) also appear formidable: well-established procedures, with very low hospital mortality rates and, in our experience, excellent long-term results.

So which is better, atrial switching or arterial switching? I think that no one knows at the present time. I also think that no one can confidently predict the future in our field. Medical prophecy is surely hilarious. We began with atrial switches because we were able to make them work. Now the pendulum is swinging in the direction of arterial switches. Why? Because we are now learning how to make them work also, and because, as mentioned previously, there are reasons for thinking that the arterial switch may prove to be superior to the atrial switch in the long run.

It is worth remembering that *the oldest known case of classical corrected transposition*, i.e., TGA [S,L,L], died at the age of 73 years from heart failure due mainly to tricuspid regurgitation (left-sided).[39] Although it is often said that "one mouse is no mouse," this case does suggest that the RV can function satisfactorily as the systemic ventricle, despite the coexistence of chronic tricuspid regurgitation (left-sided). So it is *possible* for the systemic RV to do well for a lifetime.[39] But functional studies have repeatedly shown that post-operative atrial switch patients typically function less well than normal.[40-42]

The systemic RV in physiologically corrected L-TGA[39] may be importantly different from that of physiologically uncorrected D-TGA. Recently, Baño-Rodrigo and his colleagues[43] have shown that in D-TGA, the RV free wall is thicker than normal from the first month of life onward. This is a fascinating and unexpected finding. Why should the RV free wall be thicker than the normal LV free wall in control heart specimens?[43] To my knowledge, no one knows the answer to this question.

However, we have a hypothesis, namely, that this intriguing finding—which may well be of functional importance—could be due to the coronary arteries' being perfused with unsaturated blood, which causes marked enlargement of the coronary arterial system with coronary neoarterialization (much new arterial formation). A number of years ago at an American Heart Association meeting there was a very interesting paper concerning switching of the superior vena cava of dogs into the left atrium. The effects on the coronary arteries, shown by coronary arterial casts, were dramatic (as above). The unsaturated blood may have dropped the coronary arterial resistance, leading to significantly increased coronary arterial blood flow and a much larger coronary arterial bed.

Did this lead to left ventricular myocardial hypertrophy? I don't think this was looked at (to the best of my recollection).

So, as far as D-TGA is concerned, unsaturated blood in the systemic circuit may reduce the coronary arterial resistance and the systemic arterial resistance, perhaps leading to increased coronary arterial blood flow, a larger than normal coronary arterial bed (as in the desaturated dogs), plus increased systemic right ventricular flow work due to systemic afterload reduction, perhaps due to hypoxemia and/or acidosis, or some other factor.

Whatever the mechanism of the systemic right ventricular hypertrophy in D-TGA may be, *myocyte hypertrophy* is functionally disadvantageous[44] and could perhaps result in an hypertrophied and therefore "muscle-bound" RV that would consequently function subnormally. The finding of progressively increasing right ventricular hypertrophy in D-TGA may well be of considerable physiological and surgical importance. These data[43] could be viewed as yet another indication for early surgical repair of D-TGA, and for making the LV the systemic ventricle.

To *summarize*, if technically feasible with a low mortality rate, I suspect that using the LV as the systemic ventricle in TGA may be preferable to using the RV as the systemic ventricle, for the following reasons:

1. Arrhythmias are not a problem with the arterial switch procedure (if coronary kinking is avoided), but are a major problem of the atrial switch procedures.
2. Tricuspid regurgitation may be a problem with the systemic RV: conical RV shape, spherical tricuspid orifice, spindly papillary muscles.
3. The systemic RV has only one coronary artery (the right coronary artery) and one radiation of the conduction system (the right bundle branch).
4. The RV free wall has less compact myocardium (1/3 of its thickness) than does the LV (2/3 of its thickness).
5. Functional left ventricular outflow tract obstruction is avoided by conical LV, but is encouraged by crescentic LV (with conical RV).
6. Diminished RV contractility is related to smallness of true

RV (inflow tract only), the presence of much hypokinetic infundibular "dead wood," and the presence of progressive right ventricular hypertrophy, which is functionally disadvantageous.

In conclusion, although I suspect (for the above-mentioned reasons) that the LV and mitral valve may be better than the RV and tricuspid valve to support the systemic circulation for a lifetime, this is merely an hypothesis that awaits proof or disproof. It is now possible to switch the systemic and pulmonary circulations at all three levels: atrial (Senning and Mustard operations), ventricular (McGoon procedure, i.e., intraventricular rerouting), and arterial (Jatene and modifications thereof). Within the foreseeable future, it seems very probable that all three types of operations will continue to be performed, depending on the precise problem presented by the patient, and the preference of the cardiologists and cardiac surgeons who are involved.

Summary

There are six main types of TGA (Fig. 1), and at least 33 different subtypes (Table I), based on analysis of the cardiac segments and the associated malformations in 243 autopsied cases. TGA appears to result from malformation of the infundibulum, not from anomalous development of the aorticopulmonary septum

Acknowledgments: My thanks to Margaret W. Stevenson for typing the manuscript, and Terence Wrightson, Michael Mantone, Domenic Screnci and Leslie Partridge for photography.

References

1. Baillie M: *The Morbid Anatomy of Some of the Most Important Parts of the Human Body*, ed 2 London, Johnson and Nicol, 1797, pp 38–40.
2. Langstaff: Case of singular mal-formation of the heart. *London Med Rev* 4:88–89, 1811.
3. Farre JR: *Pathologic Researches. I. On Malformations of the Human Heart: Illustrated by numerous cases, and five plates, containing fourteen figures; and preceded by some observations on the method of improving the diagnostic part of*

medicine. London, Longman, Hurst, Rees, Orme and Brown, 1814, pp 28–31.

4. Von Rokitansky CF: *Die Defect Der Scheidewande Des Herzens*. Vienna, Braumuller, 1875, pp 78–89.

5. Vierordt H: Die angeborenen herzkrankheiten. In H Vierordt (ed), *Nothnagel's Spez Path Therapie*, Vienna, Alfred Hölder, 1898, vol 15, pp. 107–132.

6. Abbott ME: Congenital cardiac disease. In N Osler, T McCrae's (eds) *Modern Medicine*, ed 2. Philadelphia and New York, Lea & Febiger, 1915, pp. 379–386.

7. Spitzer A: *The Architecture of Normal and Malformed Hearts. A Phylogenetic Theory of Their Development*, Lev M, Vass A (trans). Springfield, Illinois, Charles C Thomas, 1951. (Translation from *Virchows Arch* [A] 243:81–272, 1923.

8. Harris JS, Farber S: Transposition of the great cardiac vessels with special reference to the phylogenetic theory of Spitzer. *Arch Pathol* 28:427–502, 1939.

9. Cardell BS: Corrected transposition of the great vessels. *Br Heart J* 18:186–192, 1956.

10. Neufeld HN, DuShane JW, Wood EH, et al.: Origin of both great vessels from the right ventricle. I. Without pulmonary stenosis. *Circulation* 23:399–412, 1961.

11. Neufeld HN, DuShane JW, Edwards JE: Origin of both great vessels from the right ventricle. II. With pulmonary stenosis. *Circulation* 23:603–612, 1961.

12. Neufeld HN, Lucas RV Jr, Lester RG, et al.: Origin of both great vessels from the right ventricle without pulmonary stenosis. *Br Heart J* 24:393–408, 1962.

13. Van Praagh R, Pérez-Treviño C, López-Cuellar M, et al.: Transposition of the great arteries with posterior aorta, anterior pulmonary artery, subpulmonary conus and fibrous continuity between aortic and atrioventricular valves. *Am J Cardiol* 28:621–631, 1971.

14. Van Praagh R: Transposition of the great arteries. II. Transposition clarified. *Am J Cardiol* 28:739–741, 1971.

15. Kirklin JW, Pacifico AD, Bargeron LM Jr, et al.: Cardiac repair in anatomically corrected malposition of the great arteries. *Circulation* 48:153–159, 1973.

16. Van Praagh R, Van Praagh S, Vlad P, et al.: Anatomic types of congenital dextrocardia. Diagnosis and embryologic implications. *Am J Cardiol* 13:510–531, 1964.

17. Van Praagh R, Weinberg PM, Calder AL, et al.: The transposition complexes: How many are there? In, JC Davila (ed), *Second Henry Ford Hospital International Symposium on Cardiac Surgery*. New York, Appleton-Century-Crofts, 1977, pp 207–213.

18. Van Praagh R, Layton WM, Van Praagh S: The morphogenesis of normal and abnormal relationships between the great arteries and the ventricles: pathologic and experimental data. In R Van Praagh, A Takao (eds),

Etiology and Morphogenesis of Congenital Heart Disease. Mt. Kisco, New York, Futura Publishing Co., 1980, pp 271–316.

19. Van Praagh R: The segmental approach to diagnosis in congenital heart disease. In D Bergsma (ed), *Birth Defects: Original Article Series*, Baltimore, Williams & Wilkins, 1972, vol 8, pp 4–23.

20. Van Praagh R: Terminology of congenital heart disease, glossary and commentary. *Circulation* 56:139–145, 1977.

21. Van Praagh R: Diagnosis of complex congenital heart disease: morphologic-anatomic method and terminology. *Cardiovasc Intervent Radiol* 7:115–120, 1984.

22. Van Praagh R: The segmental approach clarified. *Cardiovasc Intervent Radiol* 7:320–325, 1984.

23. Van Praagh R, Ongley PA, Swan HJC: Anatomic types of single or common ventricle in man. Morphologic and geometric aspects of 60 necropsied cases. *Am J Cardiol* 13:367–386, 1964.

24. Van Praagh R, Van Praagh S, Vlad P, et al.: Diagnosis of the anatomic types of congenital dextrocardia. *Am J Cardiol* 15:234–247, 1965.

25. Van Praagh R, Van Praagh S, Vlad P, et al.: Diagnosis of the anatomic types of single or common ventricle. *Am J Cardiol* 15:345–366, 1965.

26. Layton WM Jr: Random determination of a developmental process. Reversal of normal visceral asymmetry in the mouse. *J Hered* 67:336–338, 1976.

27. Okamoto N, Satow Y, Hidaka N, et al.: Anomalous development of the conotruncus in neutron-irradiated rats. In R Van Praagh, A Takao (eds), *Etiology and Morphogenesis of Congenital Heart Disease*. Mt. Kisco, New York, Futura Publishing Co., 1980, pp 195–214.

28. Shinebourne EA, Macartney JF, Anderson RH: Sequential chamber localization: logical approach to diagnosis in congenital heart disease. *Br Heart J* 38:327–340, 1976.

29. Tynan MJ, Becker AE, Macartney FJ, et al.: Nomenclature and classification of congenital heart disease. *Br Heart J* 41:544–553, 1979.

30. Keith A: The Hunterian lectures on malformations of the heart. *Lancet* 7:359–363, 1909 (August).

31. Van Praagh R, Van Praagh S: Isolated ventricular inversion, a consideration of the morphogenesis, definition and diagnosis of nontransposed and transposed great arteries. *Am J Cardiol* 17:395–406, 1966.

32. Van Praagh R, Van Praagh S: Anatomically corrected transposition of the great arteries. *Br Heart J* 29:112–119, 1967.

33. Van Praagh R, Durnin RE, Jockin H, et al.: Anatomically corrected malposition of the great arteries [S,D,L]. *Circulation* 51:20–31, 1975.

34. Van Praagh R, Weinberg PM: Double outlet left ventricle. In FH Adams, GC Emmanouilides (eds), *Moss' Heart Disease in Infants, Children and Adolescents*, ed 3. Baltimore, Williams & Wilkins, 1983, pp 370–385.

35. Layton WM: Heart malformations in mice homozygous for a gene causing situs inversus. In G Rosenquist, D Bergsma (eds), *Morphogenesis and Malformation of the Cardiovascular System*. New York, Alan R. Liss for the National Foundation-March of Dimes, 1980, 14:277–293.

36. Jatene AD, Foutes VF, Paulista PP, et al.: Anatomic correction of

transposition of the great vessels. *J Thorac Cardiovasc Surg* 72:364–368, 1976.

37. McGoon DC: Intraventricular repair of transposition of the great arteries. *J Thorac Cardiovasc Surg* 64:430–434, 1972.

38. Yacoub M, Keck E, Radley-Smith R: An evaluation of one and two stage anatomic correction of simple transposition of the great arteries. *Circulation* 68(suppl III):48, 1983.

39. Lieberson AD, Schumacher RR, Childress RH, et al.: Corrected transposition of the great vessels in a 73-year-old man. *Circulation* 39:96–100, 1969.

40. Graham TP Jr, Atwood GF, Boucek RJ Jr, et al: Right heart volume characteristics in transposition of the great arteries. *Circulation* 51:881–889, 1975.

41. Graham TP Jr, Atwood GF, Boucek RJ Jr, et al.: Abnormalities of right ventricular function following Mustard's operation for transposition of the great arteries. *Circulation* 52:678–684, 1975.

42. Jarmakani JMM, Canent RV: Preoperative and postoperative right ventricular function in children with transposition of the great vessels. *Circulation* 50(suppl II):39–45, 1974.

43. Baño-Rodrigo A, Quero-Jiménez M, Moreno-Granado F, et al.: Wall thickness of ventricular chambers in transposition of the great arteries. Surgical implications. *J Thorac Cardiovasc Surg* 79:592–597, 1980.

44. Hoshino T, Fujiwara H, Kawai C, et al.: Myocardial fiber diameter and regional distribution in the ventricular wall of normal adult hearts, hypertensive hearts, and hearts with hypertrophic cardiomyopathy. *Circulation* 67:1109–1116, 1983.

CHAPTER 9

Pathophysiology of Transposition Complex

James E. Lock, M.D.

Infants and children with uncorrected transposition of the great arteries (TGA) shoulder the burden of a number of hemodynamic loads. Because their systemic and pulmonary circulations exist in parallel rather than in series, they are cyanotic, have increased pulmonary blood flow, and their right ventricles pump blood at systemic pressure. A decade ago, the challenge facing cardiologists and surgeons was to reduce cyanosis sufficiently to allow the child to eventually undergo definitive surgical repair. In 1986, we have begun to recognize that the major clinical problems faced by these children are the late effects of long-standing cyanosis, increased pulmonary blood flow, and right ventricular hypertension.

Cyanosis

The extent to which these infants are cyanosed depends on a large number of factors: the size of the communications between their atria, ventricles, and great vessels; the compliances of atrial and ventricular chambers; the resistances of systemic and pulmonary vascular beds, and others. In any of these circumstances, the level of cyanosis generally is severe.

Evidence is mounting that cyanosis early in life can have long-standing detrimental effects. Several workers have noted that cyanosis will impair ventricular function, not only in transposition but also in tricuspid atresia and tetralogy of Fallot. More recently, Borow and his colleagues, using relatively sophisticated methods of testing ventricular function, have reported that long-standing cyanosis will produce apparently permanent left ventricular dysfunc-

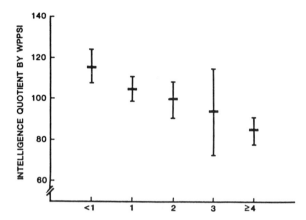

Figure 1. *Relationship between I.Q. and age at venous repair of transposition of the great arteries. (Reprinted with permission of Newburger et al.[2])*

tion in children with tetralogy of Fallot, a finding that is absent when surgical correction is undertaken early in life.[1] Thus, several years of cyanosis may permanently impair ventricular function in children with transposition of the great arteries.

More recently, similar concerns have been raised about late neurological function in cyanosed children. The observation that cyanotic children may have severe encephalomalacia is an old one. Many years of cyanosis were thought necessary for its appearance. However, Newburger and her colleagues have recently reported that psychological function, including intelligence quotient (Fig. 1) can be impaired by just one year of cyanosis.[2]

Pulmonary Blood Flow

Although pulmonary blood flow is probably increased in TGA, the precise magnitude of this increase is uncertain. Estimation of pulmonary blood flow in these children is complicated by the fact that the A-V O_2 difference is narrow, the O_2 consumption may be depressed, and the pulmonary arterial saturation, as measured in the main pulmonary artery, may not be the O_2 saturation that is reaching the capillary bed; systemic pulmonary artery collaterals from the aorta are known to be enlarged in TGA and may alter considerably the calculated pulmonary blood flow.[3]

Of more importance, this apparently increased pulmonary blood flow clearly increases the risk of pulmonary vascular disease, and Newfeld et al. have estimated that 15% of infants with TGA and intact septum will have grade III changes or higher by one year of age.[4]

The cause for this accelerated development of pulmonary vascular disease in TGA is unknown. Most authors have attributed its development to "hypoxemia" and associated pulmonary vasoconstriction. However, recent studies by basic physiologists have indicated that it is *alveolar* hypoxia that, for the most part, effects pulmonary vasospasm, and that arterial hypoxemia has little impact on pulmonary arterial pressure.[5]

A more likely possibility is that cyanosis, which is known to activate certain parts of the clotting system, causes an ongoing low grade intravascular clotting process. This hypothesis, first suggested by the observation of large platelets in cyanotic children, was given credence by the report that cyanotic children have chemical evidence for low-grade disseminated intravascular coagulation (D.I.C.).[6] In such circumstances, platelet activation may cause chronic release of thromboxanes and other compounds that serve to cause smooth muscle spasm and intimal damage. These observations should stimulate cardiologists to consider chronic antiplatelet therapy in all unoperated children with cyanotic heart disease, in an attempt to preserve pulmonary vascular microanatomy.

Ventricular Function

In addition to the ventricular dysfunction that may result from cyanosis, the ability of the right ventricle to sustain a systemic pressure load for a lifetime has remained suspect. Although it is difficult to separate out all factors that may adversely affect ventricular function in these children, the recent observation that very early surgery can restore myocardial function to normal in tetralogy and ventricular septal defect, but not in TGA, has provided powerful support to the notion that the right ventricle is an inherently inefficient high pressure pump.[7] To provide the final test of this hypothesis, several centers have begun arterial switches on neonates in an attempt to restore myocardial function in these infants. Prelim-

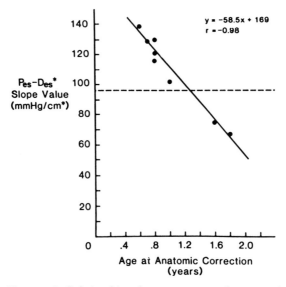

Figure 2. *Relationship between age of anatomic correction and a load-independent estimate of ventricular function. (Reprinted with permission, Borow et al.[8])*

inary data, however, support the notion that an early arterial switch can preserve ventricular function (Fig. 2).[8]

References

1. Borow KM, Green LH, Castaneda AR, et al: Left ventricular function after repair of tetralogy of Fallot and its relationship to age at surgery. *Circulation* 61:1150–1158, 1980.
2. Newburger JW, Silbert AR, Buckley LP, et al: Cognitive function and age at repair of transposition of the great arteries in children. *N Engl J Med* 310:1495–1499, 1984.
3. Lakier JB, Stanger P, Heymann MA, et al: Early onset of pulmonary vascular obstruction in patients with aortopulmonary transposition and intact ventricular septum. *Circulation* 51:875–880, 1975.
4. Newfeld EA, Paul MH. Muster AJ: Pulmonary vascular disease in transposition of the great vessels and intact ventricular septum. *Circulation* 59:525, 1979.
5. Fishman AP: Hypoxia on the pulmonary circulation. How and where it acts. *Circ Res* 38:221–231, 1976.

6. Suarez CR, Griffin A, Ow P, et al: Hemostatic disorders in children with cyanotic congenital heart disease. *Pediatr Res* 18:130A, 1984.
7. Borow KM, Keane JF, Castaneda AR, et al: Systemic ventricular function in patients with tetralogy of Fallot, ventricular septal defect and transposition of the great arteries repaired during infancy. *Circulation* 64:878–885, 1981.
8. Borow KM, Arensman FW, Webb C, et al: Assessment of left ventricular contractile state after anatomic correction of transposition of the great arteries. *Circulation* 69:106–112, 1984.

CHAPTER 10

Surgical Management of Transposition Complex in Early Infancy

Kevin Turley, M.D.

The introduction of percutaneous balloon atrial septostomy by Rashkind in 1966 drastically altered the results of therapy of transposition complex in early infancy.[1] Prior to that, the only option available in the neonate was the surgical septectomy devised by Blalock and Hanlon.[2] Mortality ranged from 30–50% with this procedure, and a significant number of failures occurred due to inadequate mixing of the pulmonary and systemic circulations. The method of percutaneous balloon septostomy afforded a palliative technique associated with low mortality and morbidity and allowed postponement of operative intervention until repair could be performed. Changes in surgical technique and methods of cardiopulmonary bypass have altered the optimal age of and approach to these patients, as repair in the neonatal period has become common.[3]

Operative techniques have involved the use of deep hypothermia and total circulatory arrest, single atrial and aortic cannulation, and avoidance of nonautologous material in intra-atrial and other repairs. Two types of intra-atrial repair have been used in the neonatal period, the Mustard and the Senning procedures.[4,5] In the Mustard operation, using single atrial to ascending aorta cardiopulmonary bypass, the patient is cooled to deep hypothermia, and circulatory arrest or low flow is instituted. A vertical atriotomy is performed and the atrial septum is incised down between the pulmonary veins, with atrial flaps developed to augment the internal baffle. The latter is constructed using pericardium, and generous superior and inferior anastomoses are performed. The area of the limbus is re-endothelialized to prevent ingrowth of scar tissue, thus avoiding superior

143

caval obstruction. The area of sinus nodes is anastomosed with superficial microvascular techniques to avoid injury to the conduction system or, more importantly, to the sinus node artery in this area. After placing the internal baffle, the left atrium is closed with a pericardial patch to allow maximal egress of pulmonary venous return around the internal baffle and into the tricuspid valve.[6]

The Senning procedure is performed using a longitudinal incision in the right atrium, once again under deep hypothermia and total circulatory arrest or low flow. An incision is made in the atrial septum in the area of the limbus, which is re-endothelialized to prevent ingrowth of scar tissue and superior caval obstruction, as with the Mustard procedure. The septal tissue is sutured posteriorly using the base of the left atrial appendage and, occasionally, a small piece of pericardium to augment it. The anterior portion of the baffle is then constructed using the free right atrial wall with the inferior caval valve forming a portion of the baffle in the neonate. The left atrium with Sondergaard's groove is then incised, with a small incision onto the right pulmonary vein to maximize the flow around the internal baffle from pulmonary veins to tricuspid valve. This area is closed using interrupted sutures in the area of the pulmonary veins.[7]

During the period of 1975–1984, of the 304 patients with transposition of the great arteries operated on at the University of California, San Francisco, 25% have been operated on in the first month of life (<30 days). Seventy-five patients underwent intra-atrial repair following failure of a prior balloon atrial septostomy, which most commonly was secondary to inadequate mixing rather than failure of the technique itself.[8] Using a method of deep hypothermia and total circulatory arrest in these patients, at a mean age of ten days, repair using the Senning procedure was performed in 61 and the Mustard procedure in 14. Details of average weight, pump time, and circulatory arrest time are shown in Table I.

Among the 75 patients there have been two early and no late deaths. There have been eight complications in the Mustard group and nine in the Senning group (Table II). These complications include rhythm disturbances, obstruction of the superior vena cava and pulmonary vein, and residual atrial septal defects. Such complications are evenly distributed among the infants, consistent with our previous studies.[8,9]

Early arterial switching of the great vessels and coronary arteries is also available.[10] The advantage of this approach is relatively normal

Table I
Comparative Data

Repair	#	Wt	Pump Time	TCA*
Mustard	14	3.4	46.9	37.7
Senning	61	3.2	36.4	29.4

*TCA = Total Circulatory Arrest.

Table II
Results 75 Patients <30 Days

Procedure	#	Mortality	Complication
Mustard	14	0	8
Senning	61	2	9

anatomic configuration, avoidance of rhythm disturbances, late systemic right ventricular dysfunction, and caval and pulmonary vein obstruction. However, this method has carried a higher operative mortality (50% in a pilot series at our institution in 1980), and its long-term results are unknown, although the potential for supravalvar aortic stenosis, coronary stenosis, pulmonary stenosis, aortic insufficiency, and coronary sinus aneurysm is of concern. Recent series have demonstrated encouraging results, and late follow-up of these patients may demonstrate the efficacy of this technique.[11,12] In patients with significant ventricular septal defects (VSD), early medical management followed by arterial switch currently appears the optimal method for repair, since VSD closure with intra-atrial repair carries a high early and subsequent mortality secondary to rhythm disturbances. For those with a very large VSD, a Rastelli repair or Lecompte adaptation of the Rastelli switch with minimal prosthetic interposition appears to be an excellent option.[13] Done in the older period (six months), these techniques avoid potential risks of supravalvar and coronary stenosis and afford anatomic correction not available using the intra-atrial approach.[14]

The available methods of repair of transposition complex in early infancy have changed drastically over the past eight years. Only long-term evaluation of the current methods will determine which is optimal.

References

1. Rashkind WJ, Miller WW: Creation of an atrial septal defect without thoracotomy. A palliative approach to complete transposition of the great arteries. *JAMA* 196:991–992, 1966.
2. Blalock A, Hanlon CR: The surgical treatment of complete transposition of the aorta and the pulmonary artery. *Surg Gynecol Obstet* 90:1–15, 1950.
3. Turley K, Mavroudis C, Ebert PA: Repair of congenital cardiac lesions during the first week of life. *Circulation* 66:(suppl I):214–219, 1982.
4. Mustard WT: Successful two-stage correction of transposition(tab)of the great vessels. *Surgery* 55:469–472, 1964.
5. Senning A: Surgical correction of transposition of the great vessels. *Surgery* 45:966–980, 1959.
6. Turley K, Ebert PA: Total correction of transposition of the great arteries. Conduction disturbances in infants younger than three months of age. *J Thorac Cardiovasc Surg* 76:312–320, 1978.
7. Quaegebeur JM, Rohmer J, Brom AG, et al: Revival of the Senning operation in the treatment of transposition of the great arteries. *Thorax* 32:517–524, 1977.
8. Turley K, Ebert PA: Transposition of the great arteries in the neonate: failed balloon atrial septostomy. *J Cardiovasc Surg* 26:564–567, 1985.
9. Mahoney L, Turley K, Ebert PA, et al: Long-term results after atrial repair of transposition of the great arteries in early infancy. *Circulation* 66:253–258, 1982.
10. Jatene AD, Fontes VF, Paulista PP, et al: Anatomic correction of transposition of the great vessels. *J Thorac Cardiovasc Surg* 72:364–370, 1976.
11. Yacoub MH, Radley-Smith R, Maclaurin R: Two-stage operation for anatomical correction of transposition of the great arteries with intact ventricular septum. *Lancet* 1:1275–1278, 1977.
12. Radley-Smith R, Yacoub MH: One stage anatomic correction of simple transposition of the great arteries in neonates. (abstract) *Circulation* 70(suppl II):26, 1984.
13. Lecompte Y, Zannini L, Hazan E, et al: Anatomic correction of transposition of the great arteries. New technique without use of a prosthetic conduit. *J Thorac Cardiovasc Surg* 82:629–631, 1981.
14. Pacifico AD, Stewart RW, Bargeron LM Jr: Repair of transposition of the great arteries with ventricular septal defect by an arterial switch operation. *Circulation* 68:(suppl II):49–55, 1983.

CHAPTER 11

The Mustard Operation for Transposition of the Great Arteries: An Overview

Welton M. Gersony, M.D.

Twenty-one years have passed since the Mustard operation was introduced for the intra-atrial correction of transposition of the great arteries (TGA), a defect which had been the most common cause of death from congenital heart disease in infancy.[1] Although the Senning procedure[2] had been described earlier, the Mustard procedure proved to be an operation that could be done successfully by most cardiac surgeons. The parallel development of procedures to maximize mixing at the atrial level allowed neonates to survive long enough to be candidates for the Mustard operation, and the result has been a dramatic turnabout in the prognosis for infants with TGA. It is a tribute to Dr. Mustard's original concept that this operation, with some modifications, is still carried out at many centers throughout the world.

Over the past decade there has been a renewal of interest in the Senning intra-atrial repair.[3] A greater number of surgeons have been able to master the required technique, and some potential advantages of the Senning procedure over the Mustard have been brought forward. More recently, the arterial switch procedure has been carried out successfully in patients with transposition of the great arteries.[4] This approach has been greeted with a great deal of enthusiasm, since the anatomic left ventricle becomes the systemic ventricle, and there is no damage to the sinus node or intra-atrial physiological conduction pathways, which result from the intra-atrial repairs.

The advantages of alternatives to the Mustard operation for the management of transposition of the great arteries must be weighed against the operative risks and long-term outlook for the Mustard procedure. Extensive late follow-up data are now available after two decades of observation of postoperative patients, whereas only recently have there been enough patients followed long enough to begin to evaluate long-term status after the Senning procedure. A significant number of survivors of the switch operation have been reevaluated only up to three or four years after operation.

A number of factors confound what one might hope to be a simple appraisal of the short and long-term results of the Mustard operation:

1. The effects of associated lesions, including ventricular septal defect, patent ductus arteriosus, left ventricular outflow tract obstruction, or atrioventricular valve deformity, profoundly influence operative results and the post-surgical course.
2. Operative techniques vary between institutions, and new procedures have become standard in perioperative management that were not utilized two decades ago.
3. The duration of cardiopulmonary bypass, the effectiveness of myocardial protection, the type of baffle material utilized, the method of baffle construction, and attention to sinus node protection are technical considerations that influence the overall results of the Mustard operation.
4. The duration and intensity of hypoxemia prior to operation may have a significant effect on ventricular function over the years following a successful technical procedure.
5. Finally, published reports tend to reflect better results than might be expected in the general population of medical centers throughout the world.

Short-term Survival

A number of reports concerning early and late survival for transposition of the great arteries and intact ventricular septum (TGA-IVS) following the Mustard operation are available (Table I). Reported early mortality has ranged from 0% to 23%; there appears to have been an 8%–10% risk for this operation at most medical centers. Mortality during earlier palliative surgery and pre-Mustard medical

Table I
Early and Late Mortality after the Mustard Operation for TGA-IVS

	No. of patients	Mortality Early	Mortality Late
Balderman et al.[5] (1974)[*]	369	17%	15–25%
Gutgesell et al [6] (1979)	71	14%	5%
Trusler et al. [7] (1980)	205	6%	10%
Piccoli et al. [8] (1981)	80	3%	4%
Schmaltz et al. [9] (1982)	43	23%	3%
Mahony et al. [10] (1982)	36	0%	0%
Marx et al. [11] (1983)	66	11%	7%

[*]Review of the literature prior to 1974.

follow-up may be higher than for the surgery itself.[6] However, a policy of (a) prompt further management if adequate mixing is not achieved in the neonate, and (b) close observation and frequent hemoglobin determinations after balloon septostomy have markedly decreased the probability that infants with TGA will not survive to undergo the operation. There appears to be little difference in mortality among babies operated on urgently in the first weeks of life as compared to those operated on electively at 6–8 months of age. Mortality for the Mustard operation was higher for patients operated on at an older age in the 1960s and early 1970s. Today, stable infants with good pulmonary-systemic venous mixing and no central nervous system manifestations at the time of surgery can be operated on for TGA-IVS at low risk during infancy in most centers.

The mortality for the Mustard operation for patients with large ventricular septal defect (TGA-VSD) is considerably higher than for uncomplicated transposition of the great arteries and intact ventricular septum. The Mustard intra-atrial repair carried out in conjunction with ventricular septal defect closure late in the first year of life or beyond, with or without an earlier banding operation, has a range of mortality reported in the literature of 20%–80%.[5,8,9,12] The realistic chances that a child with transposition of the great arteries and a large ventricular septal defect will survive through the various procedures that he or she must undergo, including atrial mixing procedures, catheterization, possible early banding operations, and, finally, intra-atrial correction with ventricular septal defect repair, is probably only about 50% at most centers.

Table II
Postoperative Problems after the Mustard Operation

Residual intra-atrial shunts
Superior and/or inferior vena caval obstruction
Pulmonary venous obstruction
Left ventricular outflow tract obstruction
Cardiac arrhythmias
Pulmonary vascular obstructive disease
Tricuspid insufficiency
Right ventricular dysfunction

Long-Term Results

Since 1974, late deaths after the Mustard operation for transposition of the great arteries and intact ventricular septum reported in series with average follow-up periods of five to ten years has ranged from 0%–10% (Table I). In addition, a significant number of patients operated on in earlier years, often when older, have survived with chronic illness as a result of persistent postoperative complications, including right ventricular failure. It might be expected, but it remains to be seen whether the more recent population of Mustard survivors will have a lower incidence of late mortality and morbidity.

The potential complications for patients having undergone the Mustard operation are listed in Table II. Some of these (e.g., superior vena cava/inferior vena cava obstruction, pulmonary venous obstruction, and operative injury to the tricuspid valve) are less often seen in recent years as technical advances and modifications of the original Mustard operation have evolved. Significant anatomic left ventricular outflow tract obstruction (LVOTO) is rare in transposition of the great arteries with intact septum, but a few cases of severe stenosis have been encountered. Dynamic obstruction, a relatively frequent manifestation, is rarely severe and does not appear to be related to the operative technique. Pulmonary vascular obstructive disease has largely been eliminated in patients with intact ventricular septum by virtue of early intervention for anatomic repair. Cardiac arrhythmias, most often of the sick sinus type, appear to be an intrinsic component of the Mustard technique. It remains controversial as to whether late rhythm disturbances of this type can be decreased significantly by modifications in operative technique. Perhaps the late manifestation of most concern is that of right ventricular dysfunction. Concerns expressed in this regard have been essentially twofold: first, can a patient in whom the anatomic right ventricle must serve indefinitely as a systemic ventricle anticipate a normal life expectancy? Second, are there specific factors in the early medical and surgical management of transposition of the great arteries that may be responsible for postoperative right ventricular dysfunction, which progresses significantly with time?

Intra-Atrial Shunts

Intra-atrial shunts via a baffle leak are common after the Mustard operation, but rarely are significant.[13] Occasionally, if a communication is proximal to an area of narrowing in the neo-right atrium, the shunt will be right-to-left and cyanosis will be present.

Baffle Obstruction

Significant caval or pulmonary venous obstruction are reported to occur in 10%–20% of patients undergoing the Mustard operation in the 1960s and 1970s.[8,14,15] The incidence of these complications has decreased as techniques for enlarging the inflow areas of the superior vena cava/inferior vena cava and pulmonary veins have been instituted and pericardial rather than Dacron baffles have been utilized.[8] Among patients in whom obstruction has been severe enough to require revision of the original Mustard operation, mortality is approximately 20% using a variety of techniques. In most instances, obstruction can be diagnosed within a year or two after surgery, but rare patients have been encountered in whom signs and symptoms of caval or pulmonary venous obstruction are delayed for many years.

Left Ventricular Outflow Tract Obstruction (LVOTO)

It is not unusual to measure a gradient across the left ventricular-pulmonary artery junction prior to surgical correction of transposition of the great arteries and intact ventricular septum. This appears to represent mild but definite obstruction exaggerated by the increased blood flow that occurs across the pulmonary valve in the presence of this defect. The gradient becomes less after a successful Mustard operation, and obstruction is seldom progressive to the degree that surgical relief of a fixed valvular or subvalvular stenosis is required.[16] An appearance of dynamic LVOTO obstruction on the echocardiogram is noted in the majority of patients with TGA and may appear to be striking. However, severe obstruction is almost never present. Transposition of the great arteries with ventricular septal defect is more often associated with significant structural LVOTO.

Cardiac Arrhythmias

The presence of sinus nodal injury in patients who have undergone the Mustard operation has been well documented. Abnormalities of sinus function and/or propagation of atrial depolarization to the junctional area is to be expected in a surgical procedure that results in incisions and suturing in the region of the sinus node and its arterial blood supply. The original Mustard procedure has undergone numerous modifications aimed at protecting the sinus node as well as atrial physiological internodal pathways. Early survivors of the Mustard operation were documented to have atrioventricular nodal damage, especially in the presence of an associated ventricular septal defect. A better understanding of the anatomy of the atrioventricular node and junctional region, allowing avoidance of these tissues at surgery, has led to the virtual disappearance of postoperative heart block in TGA as well as in other congenital heart defects.

Atrial rhythm disturbances of various types have been reported at hospital discharge following the Mustard operation in from 4%–62% of patients.[17–21] Fewer early postoperative arrhythmias have occurred as techniques for performing the Mustard operation have improved, but few published reports have included systematic long-term follow-up observation. At our institution, the incidence of atrial dysrhythmias has remained relatively constant over the years despite modifications in operative technique. A study at Columbia-Presbyterian Medical Center documented an increasing incidence of late onset atrial rhythm disturbance each year after the original operation in 76 patients.[18] Cumulative percentage of patients with arrhythmias reached 75% by the sixth year of follow-up. These clinical results might be predicted from electrophysiologic studies by Vetter and Horowitz,[22,23] as well as Gillette and his associates,[24] which indicate that virtually all postoperative Mustard patients have significant electrophysiologic abnormalities related to sinoatrial block or intra-atrial conduction. Aside from the Mustard operation itself, there appear to be no specific risk factors related to the actual development of an arrhythmia such as age at operation, type of patch, or previous Blalock-Hanlon procedure.[18] It is important to emphasize that serial 24-hour electrocardiographic studies are required to determine the true incidence of late arrhythmias in these patients. Reports utilizing retrospective data from random standard electrocardiograms significantly underestimate the true incidence of this complication.

Junctional rhythm with bradycardia is the most common arrhythmia resulting from the Mustard operation. Tachyarrhythmias occur within the context of tachycardia/bradycardia syndrome. Bradycardia is generally well tolerated and pacemaker insertion is rarely required. In our series, 8% of the patients, all of whom are alive, have required pacemaker insertion on the basis of one or more of the following criteria: (1) heart rate less than 30 per minute, (2) Stokes-Adams episodes, (3) need for pharmacologic management of tachyarrhythmia using agents other than digitalis, and (4) poor ventricular function with bradycardia, especially with documented ventricular ectopic activity.

Sudden death may occur secondary to documented or apparent rhythm disturbances after the Mustard operation, but this is relatively rare—only 3% in the Columbia series.

Pulmonary Vascular Disease

Pathological studies of the lungs at postmortem examination of infants with transposition of the great arteries with intact ventricular septum have shown significant pulmonary vascular disease at one year of age.[25,26] However, a Mustard procedure carried out prior to the end of the first year of life in a patient with TGA-IVS virtually eliminates the possibility of clinical pulmonary vascular obstructive disease as a late complication. Patients with documented low pulmonary vascular resistance prior to the age of one year and who have undergone an intra-atrial switch procedure have normal pulmonary artery pressure when catheterized years after surgery.[6,8,10,11]

Medial and intimal vasular changes are more severe and occur earlier among infants with transposition of the great arteries with ventricular septal defect and pulmonary artery hypertension.[25,26] These patients may show signs of pulmonary vascular obstructive disease as early as six months of age. This complication occurs in a significant number of patients in whom pulmonary artery banding or correction is delayed beyond this age, even if a successful repair procedure is carried out later in the first year of life. Pulmonary vascular obstructive disease is an expected late manifestation in patients with TGA-VSD operated on beyond 12–18 months of age.

Right Ventricular Dysfunction

Abnormal right ventricular performance is a relatively common long-term manifestation in patients who have had a technically successful Mustard operation.[27–30] Evaluation for minimal abnormalities in right ventricular function has been possible only in recent years as echocardiographic and radionuclide techniques have become more reliable. There are a number of potential explanations for this phenomenon: (1) surgical damage to the tricuspid valve, a complication rarely encountered in the present era; (2) effects on myocardial performance of long-standing severe hypoxemia, especially in patients operated on at a later than optimal age; (3) failure of intraoperative myocardial protection.

Recent studies have suggested that right ventricular performance appears to be far better among patients who have been operated on more recently at a younger age, who have not had severe chronic hypoxemia, and in whom intraoperative myocardial protection appears to have been optimal.[29,30] However, laboratory evidence of mild right ventricular dysfunction and suboptimal performance on exercise studies still can be demonstrated in the majority of patients after intra-atrial correction.[30–32] The effect of mild right ventricular dysfunction on life expectancy is unknown.

Summary

It appears that in established medical centers more than 85% of patients with TGA-IVS can be expected to be long-term survivors of the Mustard operation. Operative mortality and late complications among patients with TGA-VSD is significantly greater. The vast majority of children with TGA who have had an intra-atrial repair lead normal lives with the exception of mild degrees of exercise intolerance. Late death occurs in less than 5% of the postoperative patients within 10-15 years of follow-up. Cardiac arrhythmias, most often benign, can be found in virtually all of the patients if followed long enough, but sudden death or requirements for pacemaker insertion are uncommon manifestations, at least during the first two decades of observation.

Residual structural abnormalities, including baffle obstruction, large intracardiac shunts and tricuspid valve injury are rare for patients operated on in recent years. Late pulmonary vascular obstructive disease in patients with TGA-IVS is prevented by early correction. The major long-term concern is that of right ventricular dysfunction. It remains to be seen whether earlier surgical intervention and better myocardial protection will result in satisfactory right ventricular performance through adulthood.

Comparison of the Mustard Operation with Other Procedures

It is difficult to compare the results of the Mustard and Senning operations. The latter has been carried out in the past decade for the most part on better surgical candidates. The follow-up period has been shorter. At this time, there is no evidence that shows that a modified Mustard operation done by a skilled surgeon would be associated with a different prognosis or complication rate than a Senning procedure. Baseline long-term information regarding Mustard or Senning results must be updated constantly as the long-term follow-up of patients who have had a switch procedure begins to become available.

It seems clear that, when possible, the switch operation[4] is now a better alternative to intra-atrial procedures combined with repair of ventricular septal defect. A switch procedure with ventricular septal defect closure done within the first few months of life should virtually eliminate the risk of pulmonary vascular obstructive disease. Additionally it could be performed at a far lower risk than the cumulative risk of banding plus later intra-atrial correction or an early Mustard or Senning with ventricular septal defect closure. Although late assessment is unavailable in a large number of patients, the relatively poor overall results for intra-atrial repair justify the switch approach for TGA-VSD.

Early results from a few centers seem to indicate that a switch procedure for TGA-IVS during the neonatal period, or somewhat later after early banding, can be achieved at low risk and can result in excellent hemodynamics.[33-35] The long-term results of this operation have yet to be fully evaluated, since there are too few patients from more than one or two centers who have survived a sufficient number of years. As follow-up data become available from more institutions, the risks and benefits of this procedure can be more realistically compared to the intra-atrial corrective operations. However, at this writing, the excellent results from early Mustard or Senning operations preclude the recommendation that all centers attempt neonatal switch operations for TGA-IVS.

References

1. Mustard WT, Keith JD, Trusler GA, et al.: The surgical management of transposition of the great vessels. *J Thorac Cardiovasc Surg* 48:953–958, 1964.
2. Senning A: Surgical correction of transposition of the great vessels. *Surgery* 45:966–980, 1959.
3. Quaegebeur JM, Rohmer J, Brom AG: Revival of the Senning operation in the treatment of transposition of the great arteries. Preliminary report on recent experience. *Thorax* 32:517–524, 1977.
4. Jatene AD, Fontes VF, Paulista PP, et al.: Anatomic correction of transposition of the great vessels. *J Thorac Cardiovasc Surg* 72:364–370, 1976.
5. Balderman SC, Athanasuleas CL, Anagnostopoulos CE: The atrial baffle operation for transposition of the great arteries. A review of 591 reported cases. *Ann Thorac Surg* 17:114–121, 1974.
6. Gutgesell HP, Garson A, McNamara DG: Prognosis for the newborn with transposition of the great arteries. *Am J Cardiol* 44:96–100, 1979.
7. Trusler GA, Williams WG, Szukawa T, et al.: Current results with the Mustard operation in isolated transposition of the great arteries. J *Thorac Cardiovasc Surg* 80:381–389, 1980.
8. Piccoli GP, Wilkinson JL, Arnold R, et al.: Appraisal of the Mustard procedure for the physiological correction of "simple" transposition of the great arteries. Eighty consecutive cases, 1970–1980. *J Thorac Cardiovasc Surg* 82:436–446, 1981.
9. Schmaltz AA, Knab I, Seybold-Epting W, et al.: Prognosis of children with transposition of the great arteries treated in a regional heart centre between 1967 and 1979. *Eur Heart J* 3:570–576, 1982.

10. Mahony L, Turley K, Ebert P, et al.: Long-term results after atrial repair of transposition of the great arteries in early infancy. *Circulation* 66:253–258, 1982.

11. Marx GR, Hougen TJ, Norwood WI, et al.: Transposition of the great arteries with intact ventricular septum: results of Mustard and Senning operations in 123 consecutive patients. *JACC* 1:476–483, 1983.

12. Penkoske PA, Westerman GR, Marx GR, et al.: Transposition of the great arteries and ventricular septal defect: results with the Senning operation and closure of the ventricular septal defect in infants. *Ann Thorac Surg* 36:281–288, 1983.

13. Park SC, Neches WH, Mathews RA, et al.: Hemodynamic function after the Mustard operation for transposition of the great arteries. *Am J Cardiol* 51:1514–1519, 1983.

14. Waldhausen JA, Pierce WS, Park CD, et al.: Physiologic correction of transposition of the great arteries. Indications for and results of operation in 32 patients. *Circulation* 43:738–747, 1971.

15. Champsaur GL, Sokol DM, Trusler GA, et al.: Repair of transposition of the great arteries in 123 pediatric patients. Early and long-term results. *Circulation* 47:1032–1041, 1973.

16. Moene RJ, Oppenheimer-Dekker A, Bartelings MM: Anatomic obstruction of the right ventricular outflow tract in transposition of the great arteries. *Am J Cardiol* 51:1701–1704, 1983.

17. Beerman LB, Neches WH, Fricker FJ, et al.: Arrhythmias in transposition of the great arteries after the Mustard operation. *Am J Cardiol* 51:1530–1534, 1983.

18. Hayes CJ, Boxer RA, Krongrad E, et al.: Cardiac rhythm after the Mustard operation for transposition of the great arteries. *Am J Cardiol* 45:430, 1980.

19. El-Said G, Rosenberg HS, Mullins CE, et al.: Dysrhythmias after Mustard's operation for transposition of the great arteries. *Am J Cardiol* 30:526–532, 1972.

20. Lewis AB, Lindesmith GG, Takahashi M, et al.: Cardiac rhythm following the Mustard procedure for transposition of the great vessels. *J Thorac Cardiovasc Surg* 73:919–926, 1977.

21. Flinn CJ, Wolff GS, Dick M, et al.: Cardiac rhythm after the Mustard operation for complete transposition of the great arteries. *N Engl J Med* 310:1635–1638, 1984.

22. Vetter VL, Horowitz LN: Electrophysiologic consequences of Mustard repair of transposition of the great arteries. *Am J Cardiol* 45:430, 1980.

23. Vetter VL, Horowitz LN: Electrophysiologic residua and sequelae of surgery for congenital heart defects. *Am J Cardiol* 50:588–604, 1982.

24. Gillette PC, Kugler JD, Garson A Jr, et al.: Mechanisms of cardiac arrhythmias after the Mustard operation for transpositiion of the great arteries. *Am J Cardiol* 45:1225–1230, 1980.

25. Clarkson PM, Neutze JM, Wardill JC, et al.: The pulmonary vascular bed in patients with complete transposition of the great arteries. *Circulation* 53:539–543, 1976.

26. Newfeld EA, Paul MH, Muster AJ, et al.: Pulmonary vascular disease

in complete transposition of the great arteries. A study of 200 patients. *Am J Cardiol* 34:75–82, 1974.

27. Jarmakani JMM, Canent RV Jr: Preoperative and postoperative right ventricular function in children with transposition of the great vessels. *Circulation* 50(suppl II):39–45, 1974.

28. Nixon JV, Atkins JM, Curry GC, et al.: Late right ventricular failure after Mustard operation for transposition of the great arteries. *Cathet Cardiovasc Diagn* 4:175–182, 1978.

29. Hagler DJ, Ritter DG, Mair DD, et al.: Right and left ventricular function after the Mustard procedure in transposition of the great arteries. *Am J Cardiol* 44:276–283, 1979.

30. Graham TP Jr, Bender HW, Hammon JW, et al.: Improved right ventricular function following recent intraatrial repair of transposition. (Abstract). *Circulation* 70 (suppl II):25, 1984.

31. Mathews RA, Fricker FJ, Beerman LB, et al.: Exercise studies after the Mustard operation in transposition of the great arteries. *Am J Cardiol* 51:1526–1529, 1983.

32. Ramsay JM, Venables AW, Kelly MJ, et al.: Right and left ventricular function at rest and with exercise after the Mustard operation for transposition of the great arteries. *Br Heart J* 51:364–370, 1984.

33. Yacoub M, Bernhard A, Lange P, et al.: Clinical and hemodynamic results of the two-stage anatomic correction of simple transposition of the great arteries. *Circulation* 62 (suppl I):190–196, 1980.

34. Arensman FW, et al.: Catheter evaluation of left ventricular shape and function 1 or more years after anatomic correction of transposition of the great arteries. *Am J Cardiol* 52:1079–1083, 1983.

35. Lincoln CR, Lima R, Rigby ML: Anatomical correction of simple transposition of great arteries during neonatal transition (letter). *Lancet* 2:39, 1983.

CHAPTER 12

Long-Term Results of Palliative Mustard Procedure

George G. Lindesmith, M.D.

The use of an interatrial operation as a definitive method of treating transposition of the great vessels (TGV) is well accepted. Significant elevation of pulmonary vascular resistance (PVR) has long been considered a contraindication for surgical repair of transposition. Our group and others have reported on the use of interatrial repositioning as a palliative procedure.[1,2] This approach has been used in those patients with TGV and ventricular septal defect (VSD) who are considered physiologically "inoperable" because of elevated PVR. To accomplish this palliation we have used only the interatrial baffling operation as described by Mustard, and have reserved the operation for those patients who have significant restriction of activity because of arterial oxygen desaturation. The intent of the procedure is to convert the patient to an Eisenmenger type of physiology, wherein an increasing cyanosis will be a reflection of increasing PVR, rather than just the result of inappropriate intracardiac mixing.

The purpose of this chapter is to update our experience with this palliative procedure, and to record the follow-up data on this small group of patients.

Clinical Material

Our total experience with interatrial operation for TGV includes 212 cases. From 1967 through 1983, we performed 18 palliative Mustard procedures (Table I). These patients ranged in age from 1.5 to 16 years, with a mean age of 7.8 years. There were 14 males and 4 females. All except one had a nonrestrictive VSD. One patient had an intact ventricular septum but also had a large functioning Potts

Table I
Palliative Mustard Patients
(CHLA: 1967–1983)

Age	No. of Patients
1.5–2 years	4
3–6 years	5
7–10 years	4
11–16 years	5
Mean: 7.8 years	Total: 18
14 Male and 4 Female	

anastomosis. All the patients had symptoms judged to be due to hypoxemia, which significantly restricted their exercise tolerance.

Fourteen of these 18 patients had 17 prior procedures (Table II). These included 11 operations to increase interatrial mixing, three to provide systemic-to-pulmonary artery shunts, and two pulmonary artery bandings. One patient had had a prior repair of interrupted aortic arch.

No patient who presented during this time interval who satisfied the anatomic and physiological criteria was denied this palliative procedure.

Surgical Technique

A Mustard operation was performed in each of these patients (Fig. 1). We have previously reported the technique that we use for this procedure,[3] and, aside from changes that occurred in 1972, it remains basically the same. In 1976, the use of potassium crystalloid cardioplegia was added to the surgical protocol. Consistently, however, the surgical technique has utilized a very floppy pericardial patch.

Follow-up Techniques

The follow-up of these patients has been conducted through review of hospital and office charts plus personal communication

Table II
Palliative Mustard Patients
Prior Procedures

Procedure	No. of Patients
Atrial septect. (Blalock–Hanlon)	6
Atrial septect. (Open)	4
Balloon atrial septost.	1
Pulm. artery band	2
Blalock	2
Potts anast.	1
Rep. interrupt. AO arch	1

with family or the involved physician. Current data have been obtained on all 18 patients and are the basis of this report (Table III). The range of the follow-up has been from 14 months to 17.2 years, with a mean of 10.2 years. Because of the small number of patients involved, actuarial data on survival have not been computed. However, at the time of the study, 17/18 patients are living. Eleven of the 18 patients have had repeat cardiac catheterization.

Surgical Results

Perhaps the most gratifying aspect of this approach to palliation of TGV with pulmonary hypertension has been the absence of operative mortality. Only one patient has died during the term of this study, and this occurred nine years postoperatively in a patient who had TGV with a VSD and minimal pulmonary stenosis. A Blalock anastomosis had been constructed at six months of age, and a palliative Mustard performed at age six years, at which time the Blalock anastomosis was ligated. One year following surgery he was readmitted for cardioversion for a tachyarrhythmia; a year before his death he had two documented episodes of central nervous system malfunction which were presumed to be embolic or arrhythmic in origin. Prior to his death he had documented episodes of sinus arrhythmia with episodes of sinus arrest, but hypoxemia had not produced symptoms. In fact, at the time of his death, the patient was roller skating.

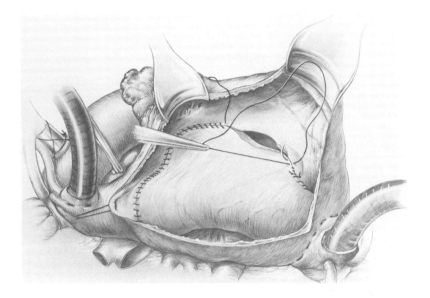

Figure 1.

It is important to note that the postoperative course of these patients was not always smooth. Eleven of the 18 patients had significant postoperative complications. It is also remarkable that they did not manifest the maximum increase in their peripheral oxygen saturation in the immediate postoperative period. The increase in peripheral oxygen saturation was not complete until, in some instances, three to four weeks following operation.

Seven patients required reoperation for excessive bleeding. Many of these cases occurred early in our experience, when control of the various aspects of the clotting mechanism was not as well understood. Six patients required ventilatory support for more than three days. One of these had subglottic stenosis of significance, and one required tracheostomy. Three patients had significant arrhythmias in the postoperative period; one required reoperation for sternal dehiscence.

Ventilatory support in the postoperative period was standard in all these patients, ranging from one to seven days, with a mean of three days. As previously stated, six patients required ventilatory support for more than three days.

Table III
Palliative Mustard Follow–up
N = 18/18 (100%)

Range	14 Months–17.2 years
Mean	10.2 years
Median	10.3 years

Table IV
Late Complications Following Palliative Mustard

Complication	No. of Patients
Cardiac enlargement	7
Arrhythmia	4
Tricuspid incomp.	3
LVOT obstruction	3
SVC obstruction	1
Pulmonary insuff.	4
Reop (VSD closed)	1
Acute CNS event (no residual)	1

Table V
Arrhythmias Before and After Palliative Mustard

	PREOP.	POSTOP.
Sinus rhythm	18	14
Junc. rhythm		3
Sick sinus synd. (pacemaker impl.)		1

Follow-up Results

In the *long-term follow-up* (Table IV), complications included one patient with superior vena caval obstruction. Seven patients had obvious cardiac enlargement, and three had tricuspid valve incompetence. One patient underwent reoperation for closure of the VSD. Arrhythmias of significance were present in four patients (Table V).

It is interesting that, in this entire series, only two patients have had documented closure of their VSD. In one patient, the closure occurred spontaneously and was evident five years after the palliative procedure. At that time his pulmonary vascular resistance had decreased to a level of 6 Wood units, and at a subsequent catheterization (nine years following the operative procedure), his PVR was still 7 Wood units. When last seen by the cardiologists, 11 years following the palliative operation and spontaneous closure of his VSD, the patient had excellent stamina and was playing basketball and other competitive sports.

Only one patient in this series has had subsequent operation for closure of VSD. This occurred 11 years after the initial operation and was performed by Dr. Ebert. Interestingly, this patient, three years after the palliative procedure, had an increased PVR from 12 Wood units to 15.4 Wood units. At that time, his PVR was unresponsive to pharmacologic manipulation. At the time of recatheterization, 11 years following the Mustard operation, it was noted that his PVR had reduced to a level that led to surgical closure of his VSD, and his postoperative course since then has been excellent. At the present time he is performing at a relatively normal level of activity.

The *physiologic data* on these patients have been based on the most recent information available.

Preoperatively, the mean PVR in this group of patients was 14.9 Wood units (Fig. 2). Following the palliative procedure, the mean PVR of the group reduced to 12.7 Wood units, a change that has no statistical significance. In this series, several of the patients had postoperative increase in their PVR, whereas one in particular (the child who has had subsequent surgical closure of his VSD) had significant reduction in his PVR.

Since the purpose of this palliative procedure was to increase the peripheral oxygen saturation, it is important to note that the preoperative mean saturation of 71.7% showed a statistically significant increase in the postoperative studies to a mean of 88% (Fig. 3). It is also noteworthy that in every instance the peripheral oxygen saturation was increased by the operation.

We have no firm data on exercise testing of these individuals, either in the preoperative or postoperative state. Our evaluation of exercise tolerance in this group of patients has been purely subjective and is based upon information gained either from the patient, the family, or the physician involved in the patient's care (Fig. 4). We have attempted to grade exercise intolerance on the basis of minimal, mild,

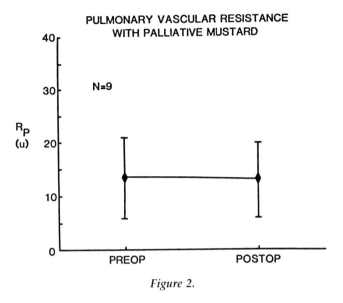

Figure 2.

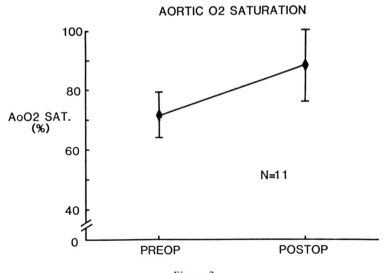

Figure 3.

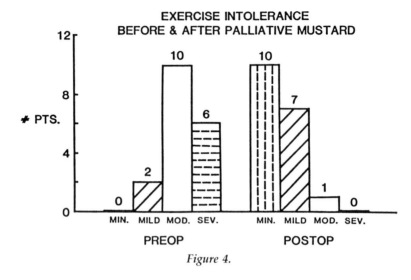

Figure 4.

moderate, or severe. Severe exercise intolerance is basically the inability to perform any exercise without symptoms, whereas minimal exercise intolerance includes those who perform at basically a normal level. It can be seen that 16 of the 18 patients preoperatively had either moderate or severe exercise intolerance, where postoperatively only one patient had moderate exercise intolerance. The others were either mild or minimal.

Conclusions

From even this small group of patients, one can ascertain that an atrial repositioning operation to enhance peripheral oxygen saturation in the presence of TGV with pulmonary hypertension is efficacious. The peripheral oxygen saturation of these patients is increased by this maneuver, and the subjective appraisal of their exercise tolerance reveals an obvious beneficial effect.

Even though only one of the patients in this study has had sufficient reduction of the pulmonary vascular resistance to warrant VSD closure, this fact seems to indicate that repeat follow-up of these patients is indicated.

Even though the ultimate fate of this group of patients is not, as yet, clearly definable, this relatively short-term follow-up (mean, 10.2

years) seems to indicate that the beneficial effects of this palliative operation are of significance in the long-term,

References

1. Lindesmith GG, Stiles QR, Tucker BL, et al: The Mustard operation as a palliative procedure. *J Thorac Cardiovasc Surg* 63:75–80, 1972.
2. Dhasmana JP, Taylor JFN, Macartney FJ, et al: Long term results of palliative Mustard's operation in patients with transposition of the great arteries with pulmonary vascular disease. (Abstract). *JACC* 3:583, 1984.
3. Lindesmith GG, Stanton RE, Lurie PR, et al: An assessment of Mustard's operation as a palliative procedure for transposition of the great vessels. *Ann Thorac Surg* 19:514–520, 1975.

CHAPTER 13

Venous and Arterial Switch Operations for Transposition of the Great Arteries

Albert D. Pacifico, M.D.

Many of us are trying to define the appropriate medical and surgical treatment for patients with transposition of the great arteries (TGA). At the outset, I will state that I am unable to answer the question of which procedure is best because, at least at this time, more information is needed. There is an evolution as any surgical technique becomes modified, and usually results improve with time. We need to review the history for each procedure, including the early and the later results over a prolonged period of time, before reaching a conclusion. Among the important considerations are the early and late mortality, the quality of life, the need for reoperation, and the cardiac rhythm.

The complications of the venous switch operation are dysrhythmias, obstruction of the venous pathways, and, later, tricuspid incompetence and reduced right ventricular function, manifestations of leaving a right ventricle as the systemic ventricle.

In 1977, we recognized problems with the Mustard operation as previously mentioned and decided to alter our type of venous switch to the Senning operation. The reasoning was to use autologous living tissue in the belief that the baffle itself had potential for future growth. In addition, the pathway in the Senning operation is relatively fixed, thus avoiding the potential unpredictability of the position of the Mustard baffle, which changes in response to systemic and pulmonary venous pressure and may later lead to obstruction. Some surgeons say the baffle should be redundant in order to leave a wide pathway; however, the surgeon is unable to control the motion of the baffle which, depending upon its final position and

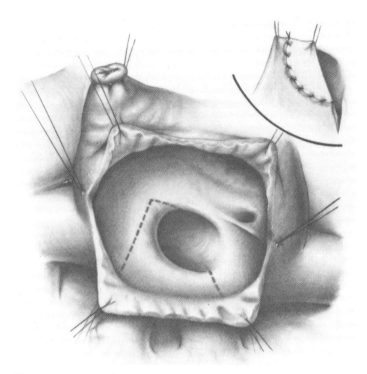

Figure 1. *Incision of the atrial septum to construct a trapeziform flap. (Reproduced with permission from Pacifico.[3])*

fixation by pseudointima, may lead to caval obstruction late postoperatively. This phenomenon is less likely to occur with the Senning operation, because the caval pathway is partly held in position by the innate strength of the tissue of the interatrial groove, and the "memory" of the atrial tissue itself, which does not become stiffened and fibrotic.

For venous switch procedures, we use two separate vena caval cannulae, placed directly into the SVC and the IVC.[1] A right atriotomy is made more anterior than has been described by Quaegebeur and his colleagues,[2] because we do not use the eustachian valve. We mobilize the interatrial groove to make the left atriotomy and extend the incision onto the right superior pulmonary vein. Construction of the septal flap is shown in Figure 1. Early in our experience, we used a small augmentation patch of either Dacron or

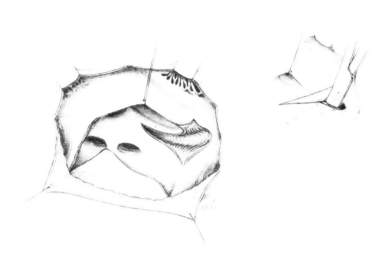

Figure 2. *Use of a flap of coronary sinus wall to augment the septal flap, avoiding the need for addition of nonviable material (see text).*

pericardium to complete the trapeziform shape of this baffle, which is then sutured above the left pulmonary veins. For several years we have avoided that by using the coronary sinus as a flap (Fig. 2). Even in a small baby it is quite significant, and its shape almost complements the shape of the septal flap, which is deficient as a result of an interatrial communication. With this method, the roof of the left pulmonary venous pathway is completely constructed of living autologous tissue. The caval pathway is completed in the usual manner. This has memory so it does not move back and forth in the same way the Mustard baffle does. The remaining objective is to return the pulmonary venous blood to the tricuspid valve. We make the atriotomy incision a little more leftward than some others do, and make counter incisions at each end. We then use an advancement technique to augment the pulmonary venous pathway (Fig. 3).

Many surgical centers have very good results with the venous switch operation. In a composite multicenter experience with 146 patients with transposition, there were four (2.7%) deaths.[3] Such results with TGA and intact septum make surgeons reluctant to employ the arterial switch operation, wondering if possibly achieving

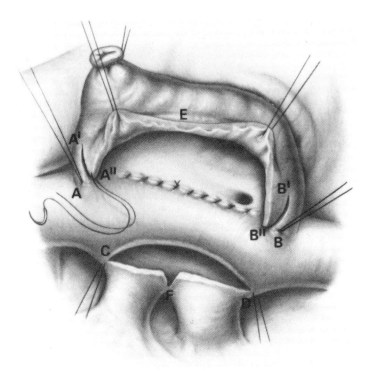

Figure 3. *Enlarging the perimeter of the flap used to roof the pulmonary venous pathway. (Reproduced with permission from Pacifico.[3])*

better *late* results justifies a higher early mortality. In the overall University of Alabama at Birmingham (UAB) experience with the Senning procedure, earlier date of operation was associated with higher hospital mortality.

The presence of a large ventricular septal defect (VSD) alone was not an incremental risk factor for hospital death in the UAB series.[4] For *late* death, however, the presence of VSD alone was a significant incremental risk factor. A parametric survival estimate is shown in Figure 4, assuming the date of operation in 1983 for the Senning repair of three subsets of transposition. Survival is similar for those with transposition and intact septum, as for those with transposition and large VSD *without* patent ductus arteriosus (PDA). However, when VSD was associated with a large PDA, there was a significant increase in hospital mortality.

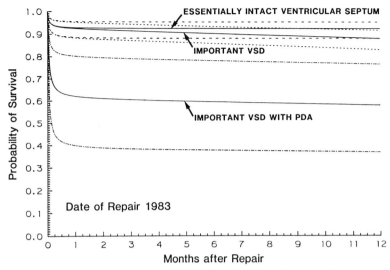

Figure 4. *Parametric survival estimates for patients undergoing the Senning atrial switch repair for 3 subsets of transposition. (Reproduced with permission from Kirklin and Barratt-Boyes.[4])*

The entire UAB experience (1967–1984) with Mustard repair included only four of 133 surviving patients who required reoperation for caval obstruction (an incidence of 3%), and no reoperation for this complication among 110 surviving patients who had the Senning repair.

The need for late reoperation does not appear to be significantly different using the two methods of venous switch. The quality of life after the Senning operation is excellent, with 96% of 103 late survivors in NYHA Functinal Class 1. However, we have no idea what it may be at 40 years.

Cardiac rhythm following the venous switch has been detailed in data from the Green Lane Hospital in Auckland, New Zealand.[4] At the time of hospital dismissal, sinus rhythm was present in 79% of patients after the Mustard operation, but in the late postoperative review, it was present in only 53%. It will probably diminish progressively with time.

An 11 year UAB experience with balloon septostomy is shown in Figure 5. Time zero is the moment the balloon was pulled through the septum, and thereafter time is represented by months after septostomy.[4] The probability of survival is stratified according to the

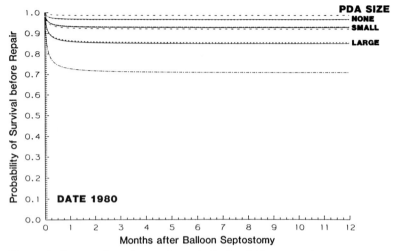

Figure 5. *Parametric estimate of survival after balloon atrial septostomy and before surgical repair in patients with simple TGA. (Reproduced with permission from Kirklin and Barratt-Boyes.[4])*

size of the PDA, which is an incremental risk factor for early death after balloon septostomy. It is evident that the presence of a large PDA associated with transposition and intact septum is associated with a very significant increase in early risk in the first three months after the moment of balloon septostomy. Some surgeons might conclude that it is appropriate to apply the neonatal arterial switch operation to this subset who are at greater risk after balloon septostomy. An estimate of survival at various times after repair can be predicted by integrating the risk (or survival) of the Senning operation with survival after ballooning in those patients with simple TGA *without* large PDA. We would estimate a five-year survival of 85% if balloon septostomy and the operation were done in 1983. Survival of 77% would be estimated at 20 years. In the same fashion, for patients wth large VSD and TGA, at five years we would predict a survival of 67%. This type of information lends support to using the arterial switch operation for this subset of patients.

Beginning in 1981, we have used the arterial switch operation selectively for patients with TGA and VSD, based on the intra-operative appearance of the coronary arteries and their suitability for switch. In 14 patients operated on during this time, it was our intent to perform the arterial switch operation, but we employed it only in

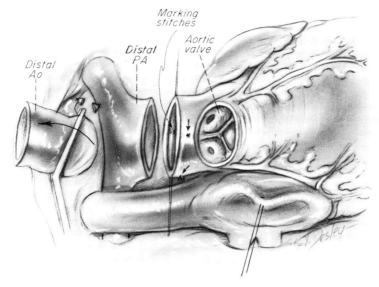

Figure 6. *The great arteries have been transected and the pulmonary artery mobilized. (Reproduced with permission from Pacifico et al.[5])*

eight patients with one death, from bleeding, in this overall group of 14. In one, we were able to accomplish a spiral internal arterial switch, and a Senning operation and VSD closure was required in five.

Our technique for arterial switch in patients with TGA and large VSD is demonstrated in Figures 6–9.[5] The aorta is divided just distal to the coronary ostia, and the pulmonary artery is divided a little more distally. As suggested by LeCompte in Paris, the branch pulmonary arteries are extensively mobilized and the ascending aorta is delivered beneath the pulmonary bifurcation and then anastomosed to the former pulmonary root.[6] The coronary ostia are excised with a cuff of aortic tissue around them, buttons are excised from the new aorta, and the coronary vessels reimplanted.

In the presence of a large VSD, there is a significant size discrepancy between the aorta and pulmonary artery, with the pulmonary artery much larger, so we have found it useful to scallop the pulmonary artery and anastomose it directly to the old aortic root, without the need for reconstructing the holes left by coronary artery excision. For patients with intact septum, this probably would not be appropriate, because there is little size discrepancy in that subset. We believe the arterial switch is the operation of choice for transposition

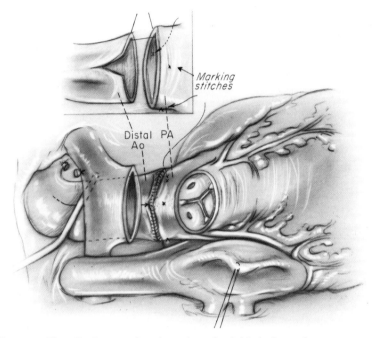

Figure 7. *The distal aorta has been brought behind the pulmonary artery bifurcation and the anastomosis completed. (Reproduced with permission from Pacifico et al.[5])*

and large VSD and continue to advise it for patients between three and six months of age; earlier if intractable heart failure is present. We believe the surgical method described is appropriate when the aorta is anterior and the coronary arteries are normal.

Dr. Castaneda has been innovative in applying the arterial switch operation to neonates with transposition and intact septum.[7] As of September, 1984, he had cared for 22 patients with a mean age of four days (personal communication). The left ventricular to right ventricular pressure ratio was 0.86. There were three hospital deaths, a risk of 14%, and to this point there has been no late mortality. Dr. Castaneda has reported that the deaths were related to problems with coronary anatomy and transfer. His experience was selected, in that some patients for whom arterial switch was planned underwent a venous switch instead due to the intraoperative anatomic findings. It may well be that with further surgical experience and refinement the

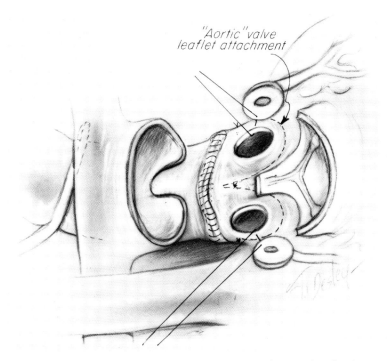

Figure 8. *Buttons have been excised in the new aorta for transfer of each coronary artery. (Reproduced with permission from Pacifico et al.[5])*

risk for arterial switch will approach that for venous switch and that it should be applied to all patients with TGA. It should be noted that new postoperative Q-waves were found on the ECG in 26% of Castaneda's series, though this finding did not correlate with post-operative ventricular performance. Eleven patients were restudied at three months of age, and the mean pulmonary artery anastomotic gradient was 25 mmHg; the mean aortic gradient was 10 mmHg.

The arterial switch operation certainly has the advantage of leaving the left ventricle as systemic, and there is less risk of significant postoperative dysrhythmia. Its disadvantages are primarily the higher hospital mortality at present and uncertainties including the fate of the great vessel to coronary anastomoses, the development of delayed aortic incompetence, and the fate of foreign material if this is required to reconstruct the great arteries. More information is needed to develop an optimal management program

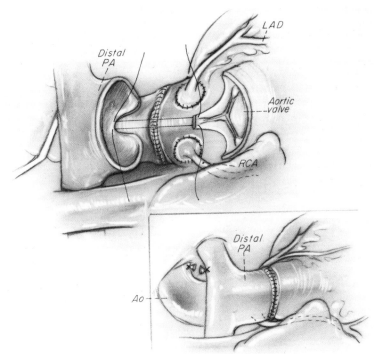

Figure 9. *The distal pulmonary artery is tailored and anastomosed directly to the old aortic root. (Reproduced with permission from Pacifico et al.[5])*

for patients with TGA and intact septum, and it must be all-inclusive. We must know what happens to an entire group of patients when they come into the hospital prior to and following balloon septostomy (if that is employed) and prior to and following any surgical procedure, be it venous or arterial switching.

References

1. Pacifico AD: Low flow bypass: The University of Alabama technique. In AL Moulton (ed), *Congenital Heart Surgery, Current Techniques and Controversies*. Pasadena, CA, Appleton Davies, 1984, pp 187–192.
2. Quaegebeur JM, Rohmer J, Brom AG, et al: Revival of the Senning operation in the treatment of transposition of the great arteries. *Thorax* 32:517, 1977.
3. Pacifico AD: Concordant transposition: Senning operation. In J Stark, M

Deleval (eds), *Surgery for Congenital Heart Defects.* London, Grune & Stratton, 1983, pp 345–352.

4. Kirklin JW, Barratt-Boyes BG: *Cardiac Surgery.* New York, John Wiley & Sons, 1986, pp 1129–1217.

5. Pacifico AD, Stewart RW, Bargeron LM Jr: Repair of transposition of the great arteries with ventricular septal defect by an arterial switch operation. *Circulation* 68(suppl II):49–55, 1983.

6. Lecompte Y, Zannini L, Hazan E, et al: Anatomic correction of transposition of the great arteries. New technique without use of a prosthetic conduit. *J Thorac Cardiovasc Surg* 82:629, 1981.

7. Castaneda AR, Norwood WI, Lang P, et al: Transposition of the great arteries and intact ventricular septum: anatomical repair in the neonate. *Ann Thorac Surg* 38:438, 1984.

CHAPTER 14

The Management of Arrhythmias After the Mustard Operation

Robert E. Stanton, M.D.

The Mustard operation is an effective procedure for the physiological correction of D-transposition of the great arteries.[1,2] However, a number of children have developed serious rhythm disturbances postoperatively, which occasionally have led to death.[3-5] These arrhythmias have been attributed to injury to the sinoatrial node or internodal tracts.[6,7] Pathological studies have confirmed damage to the sinus node and/or sinus node artery. The purpose of this chapter is to review our experience with the Mustard operation for D-transposition of the great arteries in order to document the incidence of cardiac arrhythmias and to develop methods of evaluation and management of these rhythm disturbances.

Patients and Methods

Over the twenty-year period from 1965 to 1984, 204 infants and children underwent the Mustard operation for the physiological correction of complete transposition of the great arteries. Their ages at the time of operation ranged from two weeks to 21 years, with a mean of 2.6 years. In 67% there were no associated intracardiac lesions (classified as "simple"), while in 33% there were associated lesions such as ventricular septal defect, pulmonary stenosis alone or in combination, as well as more complex lesions; these have been classified as "complex." A palliative Mustard procedure was carried out in 18 of the children with complex lesions.

There were 21 surgical deaths for an overall operative mortality rate of 10.3%, and 13 late deaths for an additional mortality rate of 6.3%. Eighteen patients were lost to follow-up within the first year following surgery and are not included in the study.

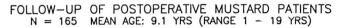

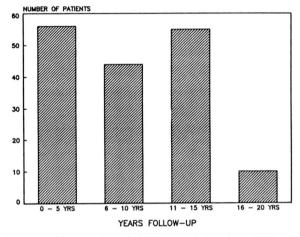

Figure 1. The number of children and duration of follow-up in five year increments of survivors over the 19 years following the Mustard operation in 165 children.

Results

The follow-up for the available 165 survivors is summarized in Figure 1. The mean duration of follow-up was nine years with a range of one to 19 years. Fifty-six percent were followed up to five years, 44% from 6–10 years, 55% for 11–15 years, and 10% from 16–19 years.

Ambulatory electrocardiographic monitoring (Holter monitoring) was carried out on 83 occasions in 61 patients. The findings are summarized in Figure 2. Sinus rhythm was present throughout in 17% of patients, junctional rhythm at some time during the monitoring period in 25%, junctional escape beats in 15%, sinus pauses in 19%, atrial extrasystoles in 16%, ventricular extrasystoles in 23%, and various forms of supraventricular tachycardia in 8%. The miscellaneous category of 8% includes first degree atrioventricular block, couplets, and ventricular tachycardia. An additional 17% of patients did not have Holter monitoring but had significant arrhythmias documented by surface electrocardiogram. These included junctional rhythm, brady-tachyarrhythmias, supraventricular tachycardia, atrial-flutter fibrillation, and atrial tachycardia.

Pacemakers were used in seven patients because of rhythm

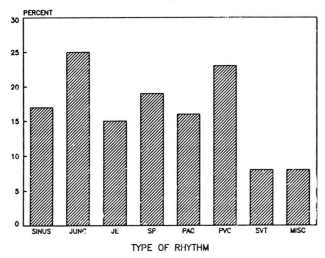

POST MUSTARD RHYTHMS: HOLTER MONITORING
N = 83 (61 PTS)

TYPE OF RHYTHM

Figure 2. *Number and types of rhythm and conduction disturbances found on 83 Holter monitorings in 61 children following the Mustard operation. (Sinus = sinus rhythm; Junc = junctional rhythm; JE = junctional escapes; SP = sinus pauses; PAC = atrial extrasystoles; PVC = ventricular extrasystoles; SVT = supraventricular tachycardias; Misc = miscellaneous.)*

disturbances as shown in Table I. There were five with "simple" transposition, and two with "complex" lesions. Indications for implanting a pacemaker were sick sinus syndrome in five and complete heart block in two. The mean age of initial surgery was 2.5 years, with a range of 16 months to five years. Implantation of pacemakers occurred from 10 days in the case of surgical block and up to 11 years postoperatively in the sick sinus syndrome. Follow-up of the initial surgery ranged from 5–14 years, while the pacemaker follow-up was from six months to 11 years with a mean of 4.4 years. Five of these children are doing well, and two have died.

There were 13 late deaths, as summarized in Table II. Five occurred in children with "simple" lesions, and eight in children with "complex" lesions, including the only child who had a palliative Mustard operation. Deaths occurred within one month to 14 years following surgery, with a mean of 5.5 years. The rhythm or conduction status at the time of death included five with known sick sinus

Table I
The Use of Pacemakers in the Postoperative Mustard Procecure

Case	Type Lesion	Surgery Date/Age	Rhythm	Implant Date	Course	Follow-up/Pacemaker
1.	SIMPLE	1970 (2 YRS.)	SSS	1979	Digoxin/Verapamil	14 YRS./ 5 YRS.
2.	SIMPLE	1970 (2 YRS.)	SSS	1978	Doing well	14 YRS./ 6 YRS.
3.	SIMPLE	1971 (2 YRS.)	SSS	1982	Doing well	13 YRS./ 2 YRS.
4.	SIMPLE	1973 (2 YRS.)	CHB	1973	Doing well	11 YRS./11 YRS.
5.	COMPLEX	1974 (3 YRS.)	SSS	1979	Doing well	10 YRS./ 4 YRS.
6.	COMPLEX	1975 (5 YRS.)	CHB	1975	Death/CHF	2 YRS./ 2 YRS.
7.	SIMPLE	1977 (16 MOS.)	SSS	1982	Death/Sudden	5 YRS./ 6 MOS.

SSS = Sick Sinus Syndrome; CHB = Complete Heart Block; CHF = Congestive Heart Failure.

Table II
Late Deaths Following Mustard Operation

Number of Deaths		13
Type of Cardiac Lesion	(Simple/Complex)	5/8
Age at Surgery	Mean 4 Years	(Range: 5 mos.–17 Yrs.)
Time to Death Following Surgery	Mean 5 Years	(Range: 1 Mos.–14 Yrs.)
Rhythm prior to death		
Sinus Node Dysfunction		5
Pacemaker	1	
Complete heart block		2
Pacemaker	1	
Sinus		2
With ventricular extra systoles	1	
Unknown		4
Cause of death		
Sudden		8
Anesthetic		1
Congestive heart failure		1
Unknown		3

syndrome; two with complete heart block (only one of whom had a pacemaker); one with sinus rhythm, ventricular extrasystoles, and myocardial dysfunction; and one with sinus rhythm. In four the rhythm was unknown. Death was sudden and unexpected in eight and was presumed to be due to arrhythmias. An additional death occurred in a young woman with residual pulmonary hypertension undergoing a dilation and curettage under anesthesia at another hospital. Surgical block with a functioning pacemaker was present in one child, associated with residual lesions and chronic congestive heart failure. There were three deaths in which no information was available.

Discussion

It is apparent that rhythm disturbances do occur following the Mustard operation; they may occur late in the postoperative period and may be fatal on occasion. Yet the number of significant rhythm disturbances seems to be less than in the past, since greater attention

Table III
Holter/ECG Correlates

Abnormal ECG/Abnormal Holter	38
Normal ECG/Abnormal Holter	25
Normal ECG/Normal Holter	19
Abnormal ECG/Normal Holter	1

is being paid to cannulation and suture placement. However, it does not appear that other physiological corrections, such as the Senning operation, are free of rhythm disturbances.[8] Our approach to the evaluation of the child following the Mustard operation includes the routine electrocardiogram as well as Holter monitoring. We believe that Holter monitoring should be carried out at two-year intervals even in those with normal surface electrocardiograms. The diagnostic capabilities of the electrocardiogram as compared to Holter monitoring for diagnosing arrhythmias is indicated in Table III. It is evident that there were 25 instances where the electrocardiogram was normal but the Holter was not. By the same token, the opposite was true on one occasion. An echocardiogram is recommended in those children with rhythm disturbances, in order to search for structural abnormalities such as baffle obstruction, ventricular dysfunction, or dynamic pulmonary stenosis. Exercise stress testing has been shown to "bring out" arrhythmias in some patients, although this has not been our experience in the limited numbers tested.

Electrophysiological studies have not been done routinely in our patients when arrhythmias have been demonstrated. Certainly, a case can be made for doing so at the time of postoperative catheterization. However, electrophysiological studies do not always elicit abnormalities such as sinus node dysfunction or ventricular tachycardia and, therefore, may be misleading as a management tool.

In interpreting the results of Holter monitoring, one must consider the meaning of "normal" in determining management strategies for these children. A composite of two studies of normal children seven to 16 years of age is shown in Table IV.[9,10] Sinus bradycardia to rates as low as 35 beats/per minute were noted, and exercise rates to 200 beats/minute were recorded. Junctional escape rhythm occurred in 26%, sinus pauses 23%, first degree atrioventricular block in 11%, and second degree (Mobitz type I) in 8%. Supraventricular extrasystoles occurred in 33%, and ventricular extrasystoles occured in 22%. Many of these same events occurred in

Table IV Cardiac Rhythm in Healthy Children N = 192 7 to 16 years	
Heart rate	35–200 bpm
Junctional escape rhythm	26%
Sinus pauses	23%
First degree A–V block	11%
Second degree A–V block	8%
Extrasystoles	
Supraventricular	33%
Ventricular	22%

those children who were studied with Holter monitoring after the Mustard operation.

Management of arrhythmias includes the use of appropriate anti-arrhythmia medication for significant active rhythm disturbances. Extrasystoles have not been treated unless very frequent or made worse by stress testing. Pacemakers have been recommended for surgical block lasting more than 10 days; symptomatic sinus node dysfunction with syncope, dizziness, or brady-tachyarrhythmias requiring medications other than digoxin; or heart rates less than 30 beats/minute while awake, although some studies have suggested rates below 40 beats/minute. Persistent junctional rhythm in these ranges may be an indication as well. The use of pacemakers in children recently has been summarized by a task force of the American College of Cardiology and the American Heart Association.[11]

Summary and Conclusions

The Mustard operation is an effective procedure for physiologically correcting transposition of the great arteries and allows for normal activity of these children. Long-term follow-up of infants and children with the Mustard operation indicates that there are a number of children with cardiac rhythm disturbances, some of which have been fatal. However, the interpretation of the significance of arrhythmias following the Mustard operation must be made in the light of findings in normal children. The management of arrhythmias following the Mustard operation includes the use of appropriate

anti-arrhythmia medication and, on occasion, pacemaker implantation. However, the outlook for children with transposition of the
great arteries remains very positive, and with proper management,
many of these problems can be decreased or eliminated.

References

1. Mustard WT: Successful two-stage correction of transposition of the
   great vessels. *Surgery* 55:469–472, 1964.
2. Takahashi M, Lindesmith GG, Lewis AB, et al : Long-term results of the
   Mustard procedure. Circulation 56(Suppl 2):85–90, 1977.
3. Clarkson PM, Barratt-Boyes BG, Neutze JM: Late dysrhythmias and
   disturbances of conduction following Mustard operation for complete
   transposition of the great arteries. *Circulation* 53:519–524, 1976.
4. Beerman LB, Neches WH, Fricker FJ, et al: Arrhythmias in transposition
   of the great arteries after the Mustard operation. *Am J Cardiol*
   51:1530–1534, 1983.
5. Flinn CJ, Wolff GS, Dick M 2d, et al: Cardiac rhythm after the Mustard
   operation for complete transposition of the great arteries. *N Engl J Med*
   310:1635–1638, 1984.
6. Isaacson R, Titus JL, Merideth J, et al: Apparent interruption of atrial
   conduction pathways after surgical repair of transposition of great
   arteries. *Am J Cardiol* 30:533–535, 1972.
7. Gillette PC, Kugler JD, Garson A Jr, et al: Mechanism of cardiac
   arrhythmias after the Mustard operation for transposition of the great
   arteries. *Am J Cardiol* 45:1225–1230, 1980.
8. Martin TC, Smith L, Hernandez A, et al: Dysrhythmias following the
   Senning operation for dextro-transposition of the great arteries. *J Thorac
   Cardiovasc Surg* 85:928–932, 1983.
9. Southall DP, Johnston F, Shinebourne EA, et al: 24-hour electrocardiographic study of heart rate and rhythm patterns in population of healthy
   children. *Br Heart J* 45:281–291, 1981.
10. Dickinson DF, Scott O: Ambulatory electrocardiographic monitoring in
    100 healthy teenage boys. *Br Heart J* 51:179–183, 1984.
11. Frye RL, Collins JJ, DeSanctis RW, et al: Guidelines for permanent cardiac
    pacemaker implantation. *Circulation* 70:331A–339A, 1984.

Editorial Comment

Masato Takahashi, M.D.

A number of interesting issues surround the clinical management of transposition of the great arteries. Some are still unsettled among the clinicians while others are beginning to be elucidated.

Arterial switch versus venous switch—a controversy in transposition. At one end of the country, a child with transposition of the great vessels may be taken to the operating room at three or four days of age and an arterial switch operation performed in nine out of ten cases, provided that the coronary artery anatomy is judged to be favorable. This is the case at the Children's Hospital in Boston. At the other end of the continent, Dr. George Lindesmith of Childrens Hospital of Los Angeles would perform a venous switch operation of either Mustard- or Senning-type sometime in the latter part of the first year of life. The postoperative results have been very good. Dr. Welton Gersony estimates that in over 90 percent of the cardiac centers in the world, intra-atrial baffle procedure remains the standard. It may be unwise for surgeons and cardiologists en masse to "switch" to a new and glamorous operation when they already have a good alternative. Although it also is noteworthy that the five-year follow-up data on the arterial switch operation are encouraging thus far, showing no late onset of aortic insufficiency or coronary artery problems, the total experience is still quite limited.[1]

The consensus among the cardiologists and surgeons who contributed to this section is that the arterial switch operation be continued to be tried in a few centers with experience under institutional protocols in order to learn more about the procedure. There appear to be a number of fine technical points about mobilizing and turning the coronary arteries at the time of arterial switch operation that might have a bearing on the outcome.

How does a pulmonic valve fare in a new role as the permanent aortic valve after an arterial switch operation?   There is a widespread mistrust of the pulmonic valve. Pulmonary regurgitation is a frequent accompaniment of pulmonary hypertension associated with various heart and lung disorders, implying that the pulmonic valve is not able to withstand an equivalent of systemic pressure load for an extended period.

Despite architectural similarity between the two semilunar valves, only the aortic valves are harvested for homograft conduits. A notable exception is the successful replacement of diseased aortic valves with pulmonic valves.

Dr. Richard Van Praagh's view is that the difference in stress tolerance between the two semilunar valves may lie in the difference in the arterial wall. The aortic wall typically has continuous elastic laminae, while the pulmonary arteries, particularly those exposed to low pressures, have fragmented elastic laminae.[2] This feature of pulmonary arteries may lead to dilatation and, secondarily, valvular regurgitation.

That the histologic characteristics which make the pulmonary artery more vulnerable to pressure-induced dilatation may be a postnatal phenomenon has been illustrated in an animal model by Dr. Kevin Turley.[3] In his experiments with lambs, effects of pulmonary artery banding in utero were compared with pulmonary artery banding in the first postnatal week. Banding performed in utero caused the pulmonary arterial wall thickness to increase at the same rate as the aorta, while postnatal banding caused the pulmonary arterial wall to achieve only two-thirds of the aortic wall thickness. The elastic layer of the pulmonary artery wall in the latter group appeared disorganized.

It remains to be seen whether the native pulmonic valve with its adjacent pulmonary trunk will be a limiting factor in the arterial switch operation and whether the postswitch "aortic" regurgitation will be related to the patient age at the time of operation.

Fate of left ventricular outflow obstruction following arterial switch operation.   Left ventricular outflow tract obstruction in the transposition may be dynamic or fixed. The pressure gradients due to dynamic obstruction are uniformly and instantaneously relieved by the arterial switch operation. Fixed subpulmonic obstructions, on the other hand, are considered a contraindication to the arterial switch operation. According to Dr. Albert Pacifico[4] and Dr. Welton Gersony,[5] similar but less dramatic changes are seen following the venous switch operations. The dynamic left ventricular outflow obstruction generally tends to improve or at least remains unchanged.

Dynamic obstruction of the left ventricular outflow tract is largely due to systolic encroachment of the ventricular septum toward the anterior mitral leaflet. Parts of the mitral valve apparatus itself may move anteriorly during systole and participate in narrowing of the outflow tract.

In a short-axis mid-section through both ventricles of a normal heart, the left ventricle assumes a circular crosssection due to physiologically hypertrophied and concentrically arranged muscle fibers, while the thin-walled crescent-shaped right ventricle is attached in front of the septum.

In a transposition heart, the right ventricle progressively dilates and hypertrophies postnatally in response to systemic pressure load and assumes a circular cross section. Limited anteriorly by the sternum, the right ventricle then pushes back against the left ventricle, which has had no stimulus to grow. Consequently, by the time the child is one or two months old, the left ventricle appears pancaked or crescent shaped while the right ventricle is circular in end systole with a measurable pressure gradient in some.

Another morphological explanation of subpulmonic stenosis is proposed by Dr. Van Praagh. In normally related great arteries, the aorta arises from the left ventricle at an angle. In transposition, the pulmonary artery arises more or less vertically from the left ventricle. This orientation makes the left ventricular outflow tract more vulnerable to stenosis contributed by other factors such as tachycardia, hypovolemia, and fibrous reaction due to impact of the mitral leaflet on the ventricular septum.[6]

One of the benefits of the arterial switch operation appears to be the avoidance of dynamic subpulmonic obstruction by stabilizing the anatomy of the left ventricular outflow region before exaggerated left ventricular pancaking occurs. In addition, it may be possible to prevent growth of at least some of the discrete stenotic lesions as the impact of the mitral leaflet on the septum is lessened.

Surgical approach to the fixed subpulmonic obstruction.   Some surgeons, including Dr. Albert Pacifico, prefer to resect the subpulmonic obstruction primarily through the mitral valve orifice,[7] while others, including Dr. George Lindesmith,[8] would approach the lesion through the pulmonic valve. In the University of Alabama and in the University of California, San Francisco, addition of subpulmonic resection at the time of venous switch operation has not adversely affected the hospital mortality. In order to determine which patients should have subpulmonic exploration, preoperative cineangiogram and echocardiogram must be reviewed carefully.

Is a large patent ductus a risk factor in transposition?   There is a feeling among surgeons and cardiologists that the patients with transposition and large patent ductus tend to do poorly. Indeed, the patent ductus appears to be an incremental risk factor in a variety of operations including the closure of ventricular septal defect in young infants. Three possible explanations are offered. First, a large patent ductus may accelerate increase in pulmonary vascular resistance due to application of abnormal shear stress to the pulmonary artery walls. Second, the patent ductus frequently causes chronic congestive heart failure and makes the patient a poor surgical candidate. And third, the patent ductus causes a low aortic diastolic pressure which, in turn, may adversely affect myocardial perfusion in the presence of increased left ventricular work. In other words, the myocardial oxygen supply/demand ratio is compromised in the presence of a large patent ductus.

Does prostaglandin have a place in the management of transposition?   As a corollary to the issue of patent ductus as a risk factor, the use of prostaglandin E in the management of transposition should be discussed. When a patient with transposition is deteriorating due to extremely poor interatrial mixing, the use of prostaglandin may turn the tide for the better on a very short-term basis. However, its continued use in the face of limited atrial communication may lead to increasing respiratory distress due to pulmonary edema. Therefore, prostaglandin should not be used as a means of delaying balloon septostomy.

References

1. Personal communication.
2. Wagenvoort CA, Heath D, Edwards JE: *The Pathology of the Pulmonary Vasculature*. Springfield, Thomas, 1964, pp 37–41.
3. Mahoney L, Turley K, Ebert PA, et al: Long-term results after atrial repair of transposition of the great arteries in early infancy. *Circulation* 66 (suppl I):253–258, 1982.
4. McGrath LB, Pacifico AD, Bageron LM, Jr., et al: Transposition of the great artery, essentially intact ventricular septum, and left ventricular outflow tract obstruction: Surgical management and results. In Doyle E, Engle MA, Gersony WN, et al (eds): *Pediatric Cardiology Proceedings of the Second World Congress of Pediatric Cardiologists, New York City, June 2–6, 1985*. New York, Springer-Verlag, 1985.
5. Personal communication.
6. Van Praagh R, Weinberg PM, Calder AL, et al: The transposition complexes: How many are there? In JC Davila (ed): *Second Henry Ford Hospital International Symposium on Cardiac Surgery*. Appleton-Century-Crofts, New York, 1977, pp 207–213.
7. Delert H, Dorst HG: Transmitral resection of subpulmonary stenosis in transposition of the great arteries. *Thorac Cardiol Surg* 27:58–60, 1979.
8. Personal communication.

Section IV

Truncus Arteriosus

The hospital, the operating room, and the wards should be laboratories, laboratories of the highest order.

William S. Halsted, M.D.

Introduction

Winfield J. Wells, M.D.

Truncus arteriosus continues to be among the most challenging lesions facing pediatric cardiologists and their surgical colleagues. This section provides the most current thinking on the subject, beginning with a complete review of the anatomic variations and classifications of truncus by Dr. Richard Van Praagh. In his discussions, Dr. Van Praagh covers the more unusual forms of truncus and correlates these with his current thinking on the etiology of this multifaceted and complex defect.

The surgical management of truncus has been strongly influenced by the excellent results obtained using early physiologic repair as pioneered at the University of California, San Franciso. In the second chapter of this section, Dr. Kevin Turley reviews the experience of that institution, stressing important technical considerations in truncal repair and providing long-term follow-up on a large series of patients.

The experience from the University of California, San Francisco contrasts interestingly with the Mayo Clinic series of patients with truncus arteriosus, as presented by Dr. Gordon Danielson in Chapter 17. The Mayo Clinic patients, having frequently undergone prior palliative procedures, provided a challenging group to deal with surgically. In a chronologic fashion, Dr. Danielson has traced the approach to repair of these patients, many of whom required complex right ventricular outflow and pulmonary artery reconstruction. The excellent long-term follow-up available for this group of patients is unique.

Certainly, the main factor in the long-term success of truncus repair relates to the durability of right ventricular-to-pulmonary artery conduits. In the final chapter of this section, Dr. Welton Gersony discusses the various conduit options and, most importantly, discusses the decision-making process involved in concluding when conduits should be replaced.

CHAPTER 15

Anatomic Variations in Truncus Arteriosus

Richard Van Praagh, M.D., Rumiko Matsuoka, M.D., Stella Van Praagh, M.D.

Truncus arteriosus communis (TAC) remains a lethal mystery—lethal because its natural history has a median age of death of approximately five weeks, and a mystery because the anomaly known as truncus arteriosus communis is far from being completely understood.[1-4]

Definition. TAC is generally defined as one great artery arising from the base of the heart which gives rise to the coronary arteries, the pulmonary arteries (at least one pulmonary artery branch from the ascending portion of the TAC), and then the systemic arteries, in that order.[1-9]

Frequency. TAC was found in 61 of 2,304 autopsied cases of congenital heart disease in the Cardiac Registry of the Children's Hospital, Boston, giving a frequency in this postmortem series of 2.6%. Of these 61 autopsied cases of TAC, 47 were from the Boston Children's Hospital and 14 were referred from elsewhere.

Classification. In 1965, Van Praagh and Van Praagh[1] proposed a classification of TAC (Fig. 1) that was a modification of the earlier classification of Collett and Edwards.[5] In the classification of Van Praagh and Van Praagh, type A has a ventricular septal defect (VSD) and type B does not (Fig. 1). *Type 1* is the same as Collett and Edwards' type 1: an aortopulmonary septal remnant is present and hence the TAC has a main pulmonary artery (MPA) component. Our *type 2* is like Collett and Edwards' types 2 and 3: no remnant of aortopulmonary septum (Fig. 1). Our *type 3* has absence of one pulmonary artery branch (Fig. 1). *Type 4* has preductal coarctation, atresia, or interruption of the aortic arch (Fig. 1). Types A1, A2, and A3 have a large aortic component and a small main pulmonary artery

199

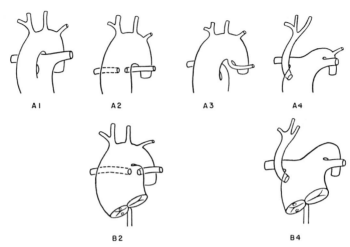

Figure 1. *Anatomic classification of truncus arteriosus communis. Type A has a subtruncal ventricular septal defect. Type B has an intact ventricular septum. Type 1 has an aortopulmonary (AP) septal remnant and a remnant of main pulmonary artery. Type 2 has no remnant of AP septum. Type 3 has absence of one pulmonary artery branch. Type 4 has interrupted aortic arch, or atresia of aortic arch, or preductal coarctation of aorta with large main pulmonary artery component and ductus arteriosus. (Reproduced with permission from Van Praagh and Van Praagh.[1])*

component, whereas type A4 has the reverse—a small aortic component and a large main pulmonary artery component (Fig. 1). Hence, in TAC, the development of the aortic and main pulmonary artery components varies inversely:[1] when the aortic component is large the main pulmonary artery component is small, and vice versa (Fig. 1).

Typical TAC. The following features are characteristic (Fig. 2):

1. a large subtruncal VSD;
2. the septal band (beneath the VSD) is well seen;
3. the parietal band (infundibular septum) is not seen;
4. there is truncal valve/mitral valve direct fibrous continuity; and
5. there are no other associated cardiac anomalies.

Frequencies of the various anatomic types of TAC:[2] type A1, 50%; type A2, 21%; type A1 or A2 ("type A1.5"), 9%; type A3, 8%; and type A4, 12%.

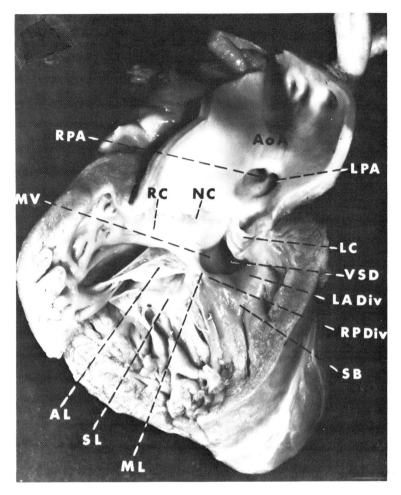

Figure 2. Truncus arteriosus communis, *Type A2.* **Type A** *indicates that a ventricular septal defect (VSD) is present.* **Type 2** *indicates that there is no remnant of the aortopulmonary septum. Opened morphologically right ventricle showing the anterior leaflet (AL) and septal leaflet (SL) of the tricuspid valve, the muscle of Lancisi (or Lushka) (ML), septal band (SB), right posterior division (RP Div) of SB, left anterior division (LA Div) of SB, right coronary (RC), noncoronary (NC), and left coronary (LC) leaflets of truncal valve, mitral valve (MV) seen through VSD, right pulmonary artery (RPA), left pulmonary artery (LPA), and aortic arch (AoA). (Reproduced with permission from Van Praagh and Van Praagh.[1])*

Table I
Leaflet Number in Truncal Types

Type	Bicuspid (%)*	Tricuspid (%)	Quadricuspid (%)	Total
Type A1	3 (7)	28 (61)	15 (33)	46
Type A2	1 (5)	14 (74)	4 (21)	19
Type A3		1 (50)	1 (50)	2
Type A4	2 (20)	4 (40)	4 (40)	10
Totals	6	47	24	77

*Percentages rounded off to nearest whole number.

The median age at death: In a series of 100 cases of TAC[2] viewed as a whole, the median age at death was five weeks. However, the median age at death varied considerably from type to type: in type A1, 5 weeks; in type A2, 5.5 weeks; in type A3, 5 months; and in type A4, 10 days.

Type A3 TAC: This consisted of absence of the left pulmonary artery (LPA) in five patients, and absence of the right pulmonary artery (RPA) in three.[2]

Type A4: This malformation consisted of interrupted aortic arch in nine patients, aortic arch atresia in two, and preductal coarctation in one.[2]

Sex: Males/females = 51/49.[2]

Extracardiac anomalies:[2] Present in 25% (25 of 100 patients). Multiple congenital anomalies were found in 14%, one patient having a C-G translocation (a rare chromosomal anomaly).

Truncal leaflets:[2] In 79 autopsied cases, the truncal valve was tricuspid in 47 cases (61%), quadricuspid in 24 cases (31%), and bicuspid in six cases (8%).

Did the leaflet number vary with the truncal type? The data are shown in Table I. We think that the number of cases in types A3 and A4 are too few to permit conclusions, and no obvious difference was found between types A1 and A2.

Truncal leaflet thickening: This was present in 66% (52/79 cases), being mild in 33% (17/52 cases), and moderate to marked in 67% (35/52 cases).[2]

Truncal valvar stenosis: This important malformation was present in 10% of the autopsy-proven cases (8/79).

Truncal valvar regurgitation: This anomaly was present in 15% (12/79 cases).

"Pulmonary" stenosis: This was found in 14% of these cases (11/79). In 10 of them, pulmonary stenosis was produced by an obstructive truncal leaflet in type A1, and in one patient with type A2. In 4 of the 11, the truncal valve was quadricuspid, and pulmonary stenosis was produced by pulmonary leaflet obstruction of the aortopulmonary window in type A1, or the pulmonary ostia in type A2. This is a little recognized but interesting form of "pulmonary valvular" stenosis.

Ostial stenosis of the pulmonary artery branches: This was found in 2 patients: in 1 patient with TAC type A3, the RPA ostium was stenotic; and in 1 patient with TAC type A4, the LPA ostium was stenotic.

Coronary anomalies: These were found in 44% of these autopsied patients (35/79). Most of these anomalies were of no functional importance, being abnormally located ostia in 28 cases (35%). However, the displaced left coronary ostium was stenotic in 3/79 cases (4%). Absence of one coronary ostium was observed in 4 patients (5%).

Aortic Arch: In 91 cases, a right aortic arch was present in 34% (31/91). Was the frequency of right aortic arch influenced by the type of TAC that was present? Here are the data:[2]

1. type A1, right aortic arch in 17 of 49 cases (35%);
2. type A2, right aortic arch in 7 of 23 cases (30%);
3. type A3, right aortic arch in 3 of 8 patients (37.5%); and
4. type A4, right aortic arch in none of 3 cases (0%).

We think that there is no obvious difference in the frequency of right aortic arch in types A1, A2, and A3.

Type A4, however, may well be significantly different as far as the sidedness of the aortic arch is concerned. First of all, when the aortic arch is interrupted, the aortic arch is absent by definition and hence is neither right nor left. Apart from this self-evident point, we have never seen a case of interrupted aortic arch (IAA), with or without TAC, in which it appeared that the aortic arch would have been right-sided had it been present.[6] In other words, we have never seen IAA ± TAC in a potentially right aortic arch situation, with descending aorta to the right of the vertebral column, perhaps because the large patent ductus arteriosus always seems to be left-sided, not right-sided (Fig. 1). In order to have IAA with a potentially right aortic arch, probably the large patent ductus arteriosus must also be right-sided; then the descending thoracic aorta would be right-sided.

If one excludes the 3 cases of type A4, then the overall incidence of right aortic arch in TAC types A1, A2, and A3 was 31 of 88 cases (35%).[2]

Absent Pulmonary Artery and Sidedness of Aortic Arch: To our surprise, we found that the absent pulmonary artery and the sidedness of the aortic arch usually were ipsilateral, not contralateral:[2]

1. Of 5 patients with absent LPA, 4 had a left aortic arch. Only one had a right aortic arch.
2. Of 3 patients with absent RPA, 2 had a right aortic arch and one had a left aortic arch.

Ductus Arteriosus: Of 70 cases of TAC, the ductus arteriosus was absent in 44 (62%), closed in 12 (17%), and patent in 14 (20%), all percentages rounded off to the nearest whole number. The very high frequency of absence of the ductus is noteworthy.

Bronchial Compression: A right aortic arch, dilated RPA, and an aberrant left subclavian artery were associated with vascular compression in one patient.[2] Bronchiectasis developed, requiring pneumonectomy at nine years of age.

Rare forms of TAC: The frequency of rare forms of TAC was 0.5% (12 of 2,304 cases of congenital heart disease in the Cardiac Registry when this study was done).[4] On the other hand, these so-called rare cases of TAC constituted 20% of our cases of TAC (12/61 cases). Of the 47 cases of TAC from the Boston Children's Hospital, four were rare forms (8.5%). *Salient features* of the rare forms of TAC:

1. intact ventricular septum, 1 case;
2. small subcristal VSD, 3 cases;
3. multiple VSDs, subtruncal and muscular, 1 case;
4. distal conal septal defect, 3 cases;
5. muscular subtruncal infundibulum, 4 cases;
6. right-sided type of TAC, i.e., entirely or predominantly above the right ventricle, 4 cases;
7. aortic atresia, i.e., left ventricular outflow tract atresia, 1 case; and
8. aortic stenosis, i.e., left ventricular outflow tract stenosis.

Associated anomalies of the AV valves with rare forms of TAC:[4]

1. tricuspid atresia, 3 cases;
2. tricuspid regurgitation, Ebstein-like, one;
3. mitral stenosis, one;
4. mitral atresia, one; and
5. complete common atrioventricular canal, one case.

Discussion

The pathologic anatomic findings associated with typical TAC are now quite well known (Figs. 1, 2).[1,2,5] However, the recent recognition of rare forms of TAC[4] has made the understanding of this anomaly more difficult and more fascinating. Let us begin by summarizing the now well documented anatomic data:[1–5]

1. TAC can have no VSD, a small VSD, a typically large subtruncal VSD (Fig. 2), or multiple VSDs.
2. TAC can have a complete muscular subtruncal infundibulum without truncal valve-atrioventricular valve direct fibrous continuity.
3. TAC can originate entirely above the morphologically right ventricle, this being known as the right-sided type of TAC.
4. TAC can have aortic atresia, which can be associated with intact ventricular septum, resulting in left ventricular outflow tract atresia, i.e., hypoplastic left heart syndrome.
5. TAC can have left ventricular outflow tract stenosis when the VSD is restrictively small.
6. TAC can be associated with major anomalies of the AV valves, such as tricuspid atresia, congenital tricuspid regurgitation, congenital mitral stenosis, mitral atresia, and complete common AV canal.

Conclusions

TAC can occur in association with a basically abnormally related type of conotruncus—with a large muscular subtruncal infundibulum reminiscent of double outlet right ventricle (DORV) and transposition of the great arteries (TGA). In other words, TAC does not always occur as a variant of normally related great arteries with truncal-mitral fibrous continuity.[4]

It must be emphasized, however, that the above-mentioned rare forms of TAC[4] are just that—rare. The usual forms of TAC and the rare forms may represent significantly *different* diseases, despite the fact that all of these anatomically distinctive and somewhat different anomalies nonetheless satisfy the generally accepted definition of TAC.

How many different diseases is so-called TAC? At the present time, we think the answer to this question is unknown.

One of the fundamental problems concerning the understanding of so-called truncus arteriosus communis is that the classical concept of this disease[7–9] appears to be erroneous, at least in part. TAC has long been thought to result from failure of downgrowth of the truncoconal septum, thereby resulting in great arterial outflow tracts that are in common, i.e., undivided. Since 1965, we have thought that this concept is at least partly wrong. We realized that one often cannot distinguish the right ventricular outflow tract of tetralogy of Fallot with pulmonary atresia ("pseudotruncus") from that of so-called true truncus without looking at the great arteries.[1] In other words, the RV outflow tracts in extreme tetralogy of Fallot and in TAC are anatomically very similar.[1]

This observation then led to the initially surprising hypothesis that tetralogy of Fallot (ToF) and TAC are closely related developmentally,[1] even though they are physiologically opposites—ToF with reduced pulmonary blood flow and TAC with increased pulmonary blood flow.

The resemblance between ToF and TAC clarified the nature of the VSD in TAC, we thought. In ToF, the VSD is not a conal septal defect, i.e., a more or less subpulmonary VSD. In ToF, the VSD is due to the fact that the infundibular septum is not where it should be, because of anterior malalignment of the infundibular septum (the crista supraventricularis). We think that this is the situation in typical TAC also: it is a malalignment VSD, not a conal septal defect in a normally located, but defective, conal septum.

Why do we think that? The semilunar valve in so-called TAC is very interesting. Usually, the truncal valve looks just like an aortic valve: tricuspid, all three leaflets of the same size.

This is very interesting because it is *not* what one would expect to find if the classical hypothesis of failure of truncoconal septation were correct. If TAC equals failure of development of the truncoconal septum, then one should have a common semilunar valve in TAC: aortic valve (AoV) leaflets, plus pulmonary valve (PV) leaflets, but with failure of separation or septation at the valve level. Is this what one sees? Virtually never. Even when the truncal valve is quadricuspid, a common semilunar valve (AoV + PV) is not present. Instead, one typically finds an AoV plus a "stranger"—a curious looking leaflet that we assume to be a pulmonary leaflet remnant. This single pulmonary leaflet in quadricuspid truncal valves is often longer and taller than the three aortic leaflets. We never have seen a patent aortic valve (3 potential leaflets) plus a patent pulmonary valve (3 potential leaflets) in common, as the classical theory of TAC requires. Instead, what one finds is an aortic valve ± a pulmonary valvar remnant.

This raises the question of what happened to the pulmonary valve leaflets. This is where the relationship to tetralogy becomes important. The question is, how can one destroy the pulmonary valve? To our knowledge, the only way that this can be done is for the subpulmonary conus to form, but fail to grow and expand, i.e., infundibular atresia. This wipes out the overlying pulmonary valve. This is what happens routinely in tetralogy of Fallot with pulmonary outflow tract atresia: the pulmonary valve leaflets are not recognizable as such.

Why does a pulmonary leaflet remnant occasionally persist recognizably as such in TAC with a quadricuspid truncal valve? We hypothesize that the answer is: the aortopulmonary septal defect. If an AP window is present, then a pulmonary leaflet remnant occasionally can persist in a recognizable fashion as such.

This, then, is how we were led to hypothesize that typical TAC equals ToF with pulmonary outflow tract atresia plus partial or complete absence of the pulmonary valve leaflets plus an AP window.[1] In other words, we concluded that typical TAC equals "pseudotruncus" plus an AP window.

Then we learned from Dr. Joseph Warkany of Cincinnati, and later from Dr. Ernst Keck[10] of Hamburg, that the thalidomide babies have been dying of congenital heart disease, mainly of two types as far as conotruncal malformations are concerned: TAC and ToF. Still later it became clear from the work of Van Mierop and Patterson and their colleagues[11–13] that the keeshond dog can have both ToF and TAC.

These three different kinds of evidence—pathologic anatomy, thalidomide teratology, and keeshond model—all support the hypothesis that typical TAC and ToF are closely related developmentally.

So we thought we knew that there is no such thing as TAC as classically conceived (or misconceived), at least as far as the RV outflow tract and the truncal valve are concerned. But we thought that the classical concept probably was right as far as the great arteries are concerned. At least, the classical hypothesis of failure of aortopulmonary septation seemed to fit type 1 very well (Fig. 1), and we assumed that it also applied to type 2 (Fig. 1). We thought that type 1 represented partial failure of AP septation, whereas type 2 represents complete failure of AP septation.

Then Beitzke and Shinebourne's case[14] was published in 1980: the heart was entirely normal, except that no pulmonary artery branches arose from the main pulmonary artery. Both pulmonary artery branches originated from the ascending aorta (Ao). The main pulmonary artery emptied through a slightly narrowed patent ductus arteriosus into the descending thoracic aorta. The ventricular septum was intact and the cardiovascular system was otherwise unremarkable. Thanks to the kindness of Dr. Alfredo Vizcaino[15] of Mexico City, we have subsequently had the privilege of studying an autopsied heart specimen of the same type.

Origin of the RPA and of the LPA from the ascending Ao is very illuminating, because in Beitzke's case and in Vizcaino's case one knows that the MPA is present.

But what if there were pulmonary outflow tract (infundibular) atresia, hence a malalignment VSD, and atresia of the MPA? Let us suppose further that the patent ductus arteriosus were "absent" (as is frequent in TAC), and consequently that the MPA also involuted and disappeared. What do you have left? This is what we call TAC type A2. It has long been assumed that because of the presence of the RPA and the LPA arising from the ascending Ao that there must be an MPA component present, despite the absence of any vestige of the AP septum, and despite the absence of any definite evidence of an MPA component in type A2 (Fig. 2).

Beitzke's case and Vizcaino's case are extremely interesting because they demonstrate conclusively that the origins of RPA and

LPA do not necessarily indicate that an MPA component must be present. These rare and fascinating cases[14,15] clearly illustrate the bipartite origin of the pulmonary arteries. The origin of the MPA, on the one hand, and of the RPA and LPA on the other are clearly separate and different. A more striking dissociation between the MPA, on the one hand, and the RPA and LPA on the other would be impossible to imagine.

Briefly, Beitzke's case and Vizcaino's case suggest that there may be no MPA component in so-called TAC type A2. Absence of an MPA component could explain why there is no vestige of an aortopulmonary septum in type A2. If this hypothesis concerning type A2 is correct (and at the present time we do not know how to test this hypothesis to see if it is true or not), then type A2 is not a truncus arteriosus communis persistens,[9] because there is no subpulmonary infundibulum, pulmonary valve, or main pulmonary artery. If this hypothesis is correct, then type A2 is truncus aorticus solitarius (solitary aortic trunk), not truncus arteriosus communis persistens (persistent common arterial trunk).

Thus, Beitzke and Vizcaino's cases[14,15] *suggest* that type A2 *may* not be TAC; but they do not prove that type A2 definitely is not TAC.

These new data[4] and new understanding indicate that it is now necessary to revise and update the understanding of TAC. *The most important points* appear to be the following:

1. It is rarely possible for TAC to occur with an intact ventricular septum, i.e., TAC type B does indeed exist. The difference between TAC type B and a large AP window is that, in TAC type B, the infundibular septum, although intact (no hole), is nonetheless very abnormally formed, either markedly shortened, or fibrous; whereas with a large AP window, the infundibular septum is normally, or approximately normally formed.
2. TAC can occur with a complete subtruncal infundibulum.
3. TAC type 2 may not be a common trunk. There may be no MPA component and hence no remnant of the AP septum. This possibility is incompletely resolved at the present time.
4. TAC can occur with major anomalies of the AV valves.

Summary

In this review of 169 personally studied cases of truncus arteriosus communis, attention was focused on the pathologic anatomy of typical cases and of rare forms. The latter are leading to a new and broader understanding of these infundibulo-arterial malformations.

Acknowledgments: The authors thank Margaret Stevenson for typing, and Terence Wrightson, Michael Mantone, Domenic Screnci, and Leslie Partridge for photography.

References

1. Van Praagh R, Van Praagh S: The anatomy of common aorticopulmonary trunk (truncus arteriosus communis) and its embryologic implications. A study of 57 necropsy cases. *Am J Cardiol* 16:406–425, 1965.
2. Calder L, Van Praagh R, Van Praagh S, et al: Truncus arteriosus communis: clinical, angiocardiographic and pathologic findings in 100 patients. *Am Heart J* 92:23–38, 1976.
3. Van Praagh R: Classification of truncus arteriosus communis (TAC). *Am Heart J* 92:129–132, 1976.
4. Matsuoka R, Van Praagh S, Van Praagh R: Rare types of truncus arteriosus communis. *Circulation* 66:II-359, 1982.
5. Collett RW, Edwards JE: Persistent truncus arteriosus: a classification according to anatomic types. *Surg Clin North Am* 29:1245–1270, 1949.
6. Van Praagh R, Bernhard WF, Rosenthal A, et al: Interrupted aortic arch: surgical treatment. *Am J Cardiol* 27:200–211, 1971.
7. Humphreys EM: Truncus arteriosus communis persistens. Criteria for identification of the common arterial trunk, with report of a case with four semilunar cusps. *Arch Pathol* 14:671–700, 1932.
8. Roos A: Persistent truncus arteriosus communis. Report of a case with four semilunar cusps and aortic arch on the right side. *Am J Dis Child* 50:966–978, 1935.
9. Lev M, Saphir O: Truncus arteriosus communis persistens. *J Pediatr* 20:74–88, 1942.
10. Keck EW, Roloff D, Markworth P: Cardiovascular findings in children with the thalidomide dysmelia syndrome. *Proc Assoc Europ Pediatr Cardiol* 8:66, 1972.
11. Van Mierop LHS, Patterson DF, Schnarr WR: Hereditary conotruncal septum defects in keeshond dogs: embryologic studies. *Am J Cardiol* 40:936–950, 1977.
12. Van Mierop LHS, Patterson DF, Schnarr WR: Pathogenesis of persistent

truncus arteriosus in light of observations made in a dog embryo with the anomaly. *Am J Cardiol* 41:755–762, 1978.

13. Van Mierop LHS, Patterson DF: Pathogenesis of conotruncal defects and some other cardiovascular anomalies in the keeshond dog. In R Van Praagh, A Takao (eds), *Etiology and Morphogenesis of Congenital Heart Disease*. Mt. Kisco, NY, Futura Publishing Co., 1979, pp 177–193.
14. Beitzke A, Shinebourne EA: Single origin of right and left pulmonary arteries from ascending aorta, with main pulmonary artery from right ventricle. *Br Heart J* 43:363–365, 1980.
15. Vizcaino A: Personal communication. September 6, 1983.

CHAPTER 16

Surgical Management of
Truncus Arteriosus in Infancy:
The San Francisco Experience

Kevin Turley, M.D.

The physiologic repair of truncus arteriosus, first described by McGoon and associates in 1968, involved patch closure of the ventricular septal defect (VSD) and valved conduit reconstruction of right ventricle-to-pulmonary artery confluence.[1] Since that time, the age at repair has markedly changed, reflecting improvement in cardiopulmonary bypass techniques and the less than optimal results of palliative procedures attempted during that period. The operative mortality has been approximately 50% for pulmonary artery banding with subsequent operative correction.[2]

The natural history of truncus arteriosus if unoperated demonstrates that, of 100 infants at birth, 75% die in the first year. Of the 25 remaining children, 35% become inoperable by age four or five, due to pulmonary vascular disease. Of the 16 still operable at age four or five, there is a 5% operative mortality. Of the 15 patients who survive operation, 20% progress to late pulmonary vascular disease. Thus, of the original 100 patients, only 12 can be expected to live relatively normal lives.

Of those undergoing pulmonary artery banding, the natural history demonstrates that, of 100 patients, 50% die at the time of pulmonary artery banding. Of those remaining, 10% die between one and five years of age and, of the 45 still alive, 9% mortality follows band removal plus repair. Finally, of the remaining 40 patients, 25% develop late pulmonary vascular disease, yielding only 30 relatively normal individuals.[3,4] Consequently, the approach of early repair was undertaken in 1974 at the University of California, San Francisco.

Physiologic repair has been performed in 154 patients under the

213

age of six months. The approach consists of valved conduit interposition between the right ventricle and pulmonary arteries to facilitate normal pulmonary artery flow and to avoid the effects of a reactive pulmonary vascular bed. The conduit is chosen to conform to the size of the infant, avoiding kinking and compression; replacement is planned with a nonvalved tube when necessary. All patients in this series had type 1 or type 2 truncus arteriosus, considered the optimal anatomic setting for this approach. This reflects the original Edwards classification, but simply refers to patients in whom a main pulmonary artery trunk or a confluence of right and left pulmonary arteries is present on the posterior aspect of the aorta.[5]

Preoperative evaluation of these infants included echocardiography to determine the intracardiac anatomy. At angiography a supravalvar injection into the common trunk is used to determine the degree of truncal valve insufficiency, the valve size, and, to a degree, the rate of flow through the pulmonary arteries. The mean weight at presentation was 3.4 kg. Since 1974, in our institution, the age for early correction has decreased from six months to six weeks. This precludes the problem of pulmonary vascular disease without increasing the surgical mortality.

The operation is performed using cardiopulmonary bypass employing an arterial line placed high in the ascending aorta or in the transverse arch, and a single atrial catheter. The flow rate has been 125 ml/min. At the time of initiation of bypass the pulmonary arteries are occluded to prevent over-circulation of the lungs. The temperature is rapidly reduced to approximately 25° C. At this time, the aorta is cross-clamped and the pulmonary trunk detached from the common trunk. The defect in the remaining aorta is closed primarily. A ventriculotomy is performed, and the aortic clamp released to allow inspection of the degree of truncal valve insufficiency. The clamp is reapplied and the ventricular septal defect closed with a continuous suture and a Teflon felt patch. The aortic clamp is then released and rewarming is accomplished while the conduit is placed between the pulmonary trunk and the right ventricular outflow tract.

Special technical points involve the removal of the pulmonary trunk with a cuff of tissue for suture of the conduit, thus avoiding distal anastomotic stenosis. Secondly, the placement of the valved conduit is such that the valve component is as far posterior as possible, avoiding compression of the right ventricular outflow beneath the sternum by the ring about the valve. The conduit may be placed into the left chest if necessary to avoid compression by the sternum. Additional technical points include a relatively large ventriculotomy and tailoring of the graft to avoid proximal anastomotic stenosis and reinforcement of this proximal anastomotic suture line with a Teflon felt bolster.

Our initial series consisted of 106 consecutive patients presenting with heart failure, 103 had decreased growth, five had cyanosis, and only three appeared normal. The mean age of that group was 2.5 months. Medical treatment was used preoperatively in 18 patients, with six deaths prior to operation. Of the remaining 100 patients, 11 died in the perioperative period (11% mortality) with equal distribution throughout the group. Three late deaths occurred; one due to sepsis, one to a sudden cardiac arrest, and one to noncardiac cause.[6]

In the subsequent period, 54 additional patients have undergone repair at a younger age with eight early deaths and one late, reflecting an increased incidence of patients with pulmonary vascular disease present from the time of birth. In the previous series of 100 patients, 88 had Dacron-valved conduits, 10 had valve allografts, and two had direct RV–PA anastomosis performed.[6] The Dacron conduit remains the most common material used because of the difficulty of obtaining allografts in the small sizes necessary. Truncal insufficiency in the initial group was present in 29 and has been medically treated in 14 with five deaths. The regurgitation was corrected by valve replacement in 24 (with eight deaths) and with valvuloplasty in two, with one death.[6]

The major problem with small conduit sizes has been pseudointimal proliferation, which is markedly decreased in the replacement conduit of a larger size and without a valvar component. The heterograft valve appears to function only in the early (first six months) period when a reactive pulmonary bed is most evident. None of the ten patients in whom the allograft valves were used has required conduit change, suggesting that this may be the most optimal type of initial procedure. There have been 84 conduit changes with 32 valved and 52 nonvalved conduits (Table I). In the more recent period, replacement with an 18 mm nonvalved conduit has produced a main pulmonary artery segment of a size equal to the adult without compression by the sternum and without significant problems from pulmonary valve insufficiency. One death has occurred in this group. No infant at the time of recatheterization has shown elevated pulmonary vascular resistance.

TABLE I	
Conduit Changes	84
Valved	32
Nonvalved	52
(Homografts)	0/10

In conclusion, early correction of truncus arteriosus is possible with a low operative mortality and prevents development of pulmonary vascular disease in a high percentage of patients, thus allowing normal growth and development. To date, no late deaths have been directly related to the truncal anomaly. Early repair results in the lowest operative mortality and highest long-term yield from operative intervention and provides the most likely possibility of a normal life.

References

1. McGoon DC, Rastelli GC, Ongley PA: An operation for the correction of truncus arteriosus. *JAMA* 205:69–73, 1968.
2. Oldham HN Jr, Kakos GS, Jarmakani MM, et al: Pulmonary artery banding in infants with complex congenital heart defects. *Ann Thorac Surg* 13:342–350, 1972.
3. McGoon DC, Wallace RB, Danielson GK: The Rastelli operation: its indications and results. *J Thorac Cardiovasc Surg* 65:65–75, 1973.
4. Mair DD, Ritter DG, Davies GD, et al: Selection of patients with truncus arteriosus for surgical correction: anatomic and hemodynamic considerations. *Circulation* 49:144–151, 1974.
5. Collett RW, Edwards JE: Persistent truncus arteriosus: a classification according to anatomic types. *Surg Clin North Am* 1949:1245–1270.
6. Ebert PA, Turley K, Stanger P, et al: Surgical treatment of truncus arteriosus in the first six months of life. *Ann Surg* 200:451–456, 1984.

CHAPTER 17

Surgical Management of Truncus Arteriosus: Mayo Clinic Experience

Gordon K. Danielson, M.D.

This review comprises a group of patients from an era and population different from the San Francisco experience. Many patient characteristics and problems are similar, but others are different. The patients were generally older, had undergone more prior palliative procedures, and had a greater incidence of pulmonary vascular obstructive disease.

The Mayo Clinic experience began in 1965 with three patients operated on unsuccessfully, all receiving tube grafts, two nonvalved and one containing a Starr-Edwards valve. It was not until September, 1967, when Dr. McGoon employed a homograft aorta with integral valve to establish right ventricle to pulmonary artery continuity, that a successful result was obtained.[1]

Repair of truncus arteriosus in patients who have had bilateral pulmonary artery banding presents one of the most challenging problems a cardiac surgeon has to deal with. The bands are put on early in life, and they usually roll out to the pericardial reflection on both sides. The adhesions are often dense, so it may be quite tedious to dissect the pulmonary arteries, especially behind the aorta. Often the distal pulmonary arteries remain small, resulting in high pressure within the conduit and increasing potential for bleeding along the suture lines. To manage the problem of small pulmonary arteries, we have often used a porcine-valved Dacron conduit opened in a fishmouth style and anastomosed to longitudinal incisions in both pulmonary arteries (Fig. 1). Because of unrestricted length in the distal portion of the prosthetic conduit, as compared to a homograft, arterioplasty techniques are more easily performed. The main disadvantage of a valved conduit is the ring stent at valve level that may compress the coronary arteries.

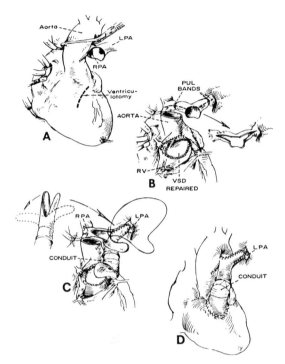

Figure 1. Repair of truncus arteriosus with bilateral pulmonary artery bands. **A.** The pulmonary arteries are detached from the truncus and the aortic defect is closed. **B.** The ventricular septal defect is closed with a patch and the pulmonary arteries are opened through the banded sites. **C.** The distal conduit is opened in a fishmouth fashion and anastomosed to the pulmonary arteriotomies. **D.** Completed repair. (Modified from RK Parker et al.[4])

An analysis has been made of our experience with 167 patients operated on from October 1965 through February 1982.[2] The youngest patient was 18 days old, and the oldest was 33 years (median = 5 years). There were many pulmonary artery anomalies, due in part to the natural associated anomalies mentioned by Doctor Van Praagh and in part to iatrogenic anomalies. Examples of the latter would include stenoses due to banding of the main or branch pulmonary arteries and hypoplasia or acquired absence of the left or right pulmonary artery. With absent or hypoplastic pulmonary arteries, and in the cases where a band has rotated so that one artery is small and the other hypertensive, the mortality and late results are ad-

Table I
Preoperative Pulmonary-to-Systemic Blood Flow Ratio (Qp/Qs)

	Banded Patients	Nonbanded Patients	Total
Qp/Qs			
Unstated	15	13	28
<1.5	28	25	53 (38%)
1.5–3.0	14	53	67 (48%)
>3.0	2	17	19 (14%)
Total	59	108	167

versely affected. One of the advantages of repairing truncus arteriosus in infancy is that the patients do not have complicating residua of previous operations.

There were 16 of our patients who had congenital absence of one pulmonary artery, and three others had acquired absence related either to a band or a shunt; 13 of the 19 patients were operative survivors. Seven patients had interrupted aortic arch, of which four were operative survivors. Sixty-one patients (36.5%) had undergone one or more previous palliative operations.

It is often difficult for us, either by angiography or at operation, to differentiate between types I and II truncus arteriosus; nearly all of our cases were one of these types. Seven patients were thought originally to have type III truncus, although in none did the pulmonary arteries arise laterally from the truncus; rather they arose posterolaterally, somewhat more distant than in those anomalies classified as type II.

The preoperative pulmonary-to-systemic blood flow ratio is shown in Table I. A low flow ratio indicates either pulmonary vascular disease or tight pulmonary artery banding. Most infants initially have a high pulmonary flow, but those with high flow comprised a minority of this series.

Of the patients studied by cardiac catheterization, 51% were found to have a pulmonary vascular resistance greater than 8 units. It is difficult to know exactly when to call a patient inoperable. Currently, if the patient is over the age of two years and the resistance is greater than 8–10 units, we believe the patient has passed the point of operability. In our early experience, we did operate on such patients and learned that the operative mortality was significantly increased.

In addition, most of the patients failed to show regression of their pulmonary hypertension and, thus, their natural history and clinical course had not been changed by total repair. Under the age of two years, there is a greater chance the pulmonary vascular disease will regress; nevertheless, some patients between the ages of 6 months and 2 years have already developed irreversible pulmonary vascular disease.

Before November 1972, the right ventricle to pulmonary artery conduits were irradiated homografts (n = 59), nonvalved Dacron tubes (n = 2), and Dacron tube with Starr-Edwards valve (n = 1). Between November 1972 and March 1982, porcine-valved Dacron conduits (n = 103) and bovine pericardial-valved Dacron conduits (n = 2) have been employed. Currently, we are using frozen fresh homografts or porcine-valved collagen-impregnated Dacron conduits (Tascon).

Truncal valve insufficiency is a progressive disease, and the problem must be addressed in many patients operated on beyond infancy. Truncal incompetence was moderate in 31% of our patients and severe in 6%. Ten patients required concomitant truncal valve replacement, and others required some type of valvuloplasty. It is difficult to know whether truncal repair changes the natural history of truncal valve insufficiency once it develops, inasmuch as some of these patients, even after complete repair, have shown progression of moderate truncal insufficiency. In this series, none of the patients under age five had severe truncal valve insufficiency. Although some patients are born with significant truncal valve regurgitation, most patients have a competent valve at birth but develop progressive insufficiency with time. Perhaps the situation is somewhat like that of pulmonary atresia, which also has a single great artery leaving the heart. In these patients, the aorta commonly dilates and the valve leaflets become incompetent as the patient grows older.

The mortality in this group is shown in Table II. There were 27 patients under two years of age. Above the age of two, the risk for various age groups is about the same, from 19%–26%. The vast majority of patients died of low cardiac output, related primarily to residual right ventricular hypertension. As shown in Table III, 45% (13 of 29) had severe pulmonary vascular obstructive disease (Heath-Edwards grade 3–4 changes), and others had hypoplastic distal pulmonary arteries subsequent to pulmonary artery banding in infancy. Other patients developed low cardiac output following

Table II
Hospital Mortality Related to Age

Age (yr.)	No. of patients	Died	Significance
<2	27	19 (70%)	p<0.001
2–4	38	10 (26%)	NS
5–9	70	13 (19%)	NS
≥10	32	6 (19%)	NS
Total	167	48 (29%)	

Table III
Pulmonary Vascular Lesions Related to Preoperative
Pulmonary Resistance

| | Heath-Edwards grade | | |
Rp (u×m²)	1—2	3–4	Total
<8	12 (75%)	2 (15%)	14
≥8	4 (25%)	11 (85%)	15
Total	16	13	29
		p<0.002	

extensive pulmonary artery reconstructions in previously banded patients.

In the group under age two, the mortality was 70%, similar to that reported by most other institutions during the same time interval. A few had an interrupted aortic arch, most were in intractable heart failure, and some already had advanced pulmonary vascular disease. Our philosophy then was to try to tide these patients over until they could reach an older age, so they "would tolerate the procedure better," and it would be possible to place a larger conduit. Great credit is due Doctor Ebert and associates in San Francisco,[3] who have shown us this logic was wrong. All that can be accomplished by waiting is to allow the patient to develop pulmonary vascular obstructive disease or myocardial damage secondary to advanced congestive heart failure. Clearly, the risk is higher when the patient is operated on under those circumstances. We now agree that operation is best performed while the patient is still minimally symptomatic and, in any case, before 6 months of age.

The postoperative mean pulmonary artery to left ventricular

Table IV
Late Reoperations

Conduit replacement only	25
Conduit replacement and truncal valve replacement	7
Truncal valve replacement only	2
Recurrent VSD closure	2

---

pressure ratio of those patients with bilateral pulmonary arteries who died was 0.53 and, of those who survived, it was 0.44 (p < 0.001). The same trend was noted in patients having unilateral pulmonary arteries. A low pulmonary artery pressure is, therefore, a favorable sign following repair and, of course, this is the case when one operates before pulmonary vascular disease becomes established.

A correlation between pulmonary vascular resistance and pulmonary vascular disease by microscopy in patients dying perioperatively is shown in Table III. If resistance was less than 8 units, most patients had Heath-Edwards grade 1-2 lesions; when the resistance was 8 units or greater, most patients had grade 3 and 4 lesions, indicating irreversible pulmonary vascular disease.

Of the 119 operative survivors, 90 are still living; 59 (66%) in New York Heart Association functional Class I, 28 (31%) in Class II, and three (3%) in Class III. Of the 29 late deaths, eight were related to reoperation. Most of the other deaths were sudden, many in patients with right ventricular hypertension or heart failure related to pulmonary vascular disease.

Late reoperations were required in 36 patients (Table IV). Conduit replacement was necessary in 32. Freedom from reoperation was 86% at five years and 53% at ten years. For patients operated on early in infancy, the reoperation rate is much higher, a fact related to the small size of the patient and of the conduit. Although repair of truncus is properly advised in infancy, one pays a price in terms of the need for early reoperation for conduit replacement.[3]

The actuarial survival curve shows 60% of hospital survivors alive at 14 years. This survival curve would be even more favorable if one excluded the 50% of patients in this series who would probably not be considered surgical candidates now because of their advanced pulmonary vascular disease. For patients who survive repair in infancy, the long-term survival is remarkably good (Fig. 2). The

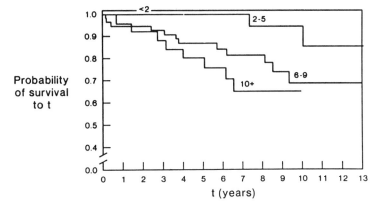

Figure 2. Comparative actuarial long-term survival to cardiac-related deaths for different age groups at the initial operation for truncus arteriosus. (Reprinted with permission from RM DiDonato et al.[2])

survival is progressively less with older age groups, and is least favorable for those 10 years and older at operation. Better late survival of young patients is probably related to lower incidences of pulmonary vascular disease and progressive degenerative changes in the myocardium. Those patients with a large pulmonary blood flow preoperatively do better than those who do not have large flow, probably a reflection of the degree of pulmonary vascular disease.

Truncal valve insufficiency is a significant factor in late mortality, those with minimal insufficiency surviving much better (82% at 12 years) than those with moderate to severe regurgitation (45% survival at 12 years). If it is true that repairing truncus arteriosus early in life will prevent the development or retard progression of truncal valve insufficiency in some patients, that would be another argument for early repair.

Absence of one pulmonary artery is another serious problem. These patients develop pulmonary vascular disease early and, even if they survive surgery, the outlook for long-term survival is poor (25% at 12 years) because of progression of pulmonary vascular disease. Truncus with unilateral pulmonary artery should be repaired early in life, but it remains to be seen whether early operation will significantly influence the generally poor prognosis of this anomaly.

References

1. McGoon DC, Rastelli GC, Ongley PA: An operation for the correction of truncus arteriosus. *JAMA* 205:69–73, 1968.
2. DiDonato RM, Fyfe DA, Puga FJ, et al : Fifteen-year experience with surgical repair of truncus arteriosus. *J Thorac Cardiovasc Surg* 89:414–422, 1985.
3. Ebert PA, Turley K, Stanger P, et al: Surgical treatment of truncus arteriosus in the first six months of life. *Ann Surg* 200:451–456, 1984.
4. Parker RK, McGoon DC, Danielson GK, et al: Repair of truncus arteriosus in patients with prior banding of the pulmonary artery. *Surgery* 78:761–767, 1975.

CHAPTER 18

The Right Ventricular-Pulmonary Conduit: Long-Term Outlook and Criteria for Replacement

Welton M. Gersony, M.D.

Considerations involved in the use of an extracardiac conduit for right ventricular-pulmonary artery reconstruction in patients with congenital heart disease include: (a) demonstrated need, (b) the availability of a prosthesis of optimal dimensions for the individual patient, and (c) the potential long-term function of the conduit that is chosen. Conduits that have been utilized include those containing xenograft valves, most often porcine or bovine; mechanical valves; aortic homografts; pericardial conduits including those containing valves constructed of pericardium; and nonvalved Dacron tubes.

Aortic homografts introduced in 1966,[1] preserved by freezing and sterilized by radiation, had a high incidence of early calcification and obstruction.[2] Later fresh homografts preserved in nutrient solution with antibiotics appeared to be both effective and long-lasting.[3-6] However, because of the poor early experience and the lack of availability of fresh homografts, and the desirability of having a "shelf" type of conduit that would be ready to use at any size requirement, most centers turned to conduits containing porcine valves.[7,8]

Long-term data are now becoming available regarding survival of various types of conduits. The porcine valve-containing low porosity Dacron conduit has been utilized in a sufficient number of patients with adequate follow-up to conclude that no more than a 5–10 year period can be expected before reoperation is necessary for most patients because of conduit obstruction.[9-11] A recent study at Columbia-Presbyterian Medical Center,[11] in which 36 patients were catheterized after a mean follow-up period of 3.3 years, indicated

225

mild to moderate right ventricular hypertension secondary to conduit obstruction in 40% of patients (RV pressure = 41–80 mmHg) and severe right ventricular obstruction (RV pressure > 80 mmHg) in 43% of patients. Only 17% had normal right ventricular pressure. The patients catheterized within two years of operation had the least obstruction, but by six years postoperatively, all of the patients recatheterized had moderate to severe gradients across the conduit. No significant porcine valve insufficiency was documented. Twenty-three percent of patients in this series underwent reoperation at a mean of 4.7 years after initial surgery.

A number of factors have been considered to be important in the chronic damage induced in a Dacron conduit containing a porcine valve. These include: increased calcium turnover in the pediatric age group, fatigue damage to the valve, and the development of a progressive fibrous peel on the inner surface of the Dacron tube. Proximal and/or distal conduit obstruction is due to this thick, partially separated neointima. Calcification and deterioration of the valve itself is also a well documented cause of conduit obstruction.[10–12] Residual stenosis also may be present at the site of the anastomoses with the right ventricle and/or pulmonary artery. Recently, knitted Dacron presealed with fibrinogen glue has been advocated as a means of eliminating peel formation.[12] In addition, experimental data are being obtained regarding pretreatment of xenografts with anticalcification agents.[13] It remains to be seen whether these new approaches will improve the longevity of porcine valve-containing conduits.

Fresh homografts preserved in antibiotics appear to have a longer functional life than the xenografts used today and often do not need replacement until the second or even third decade following initial placement.[6] Homografts, however preserved, tend to calcify rapidly.[14] However, calcification does not appear to interfere with function in the great majority of patients in whom fresh homografts have been used, at least in the first decade following surgery.[4,6] Recently there has been more general availability of aortic homografts prepared and preserved in antibiotic solution, and it appears that soon there will be a sufficient number more readily obtainable in various sizes for general use.

Pericardial conduits and mechanical valve-containing conduits have had insufficient numbers utilized and too few years of follow-up to make an accurate comparison with xenografts and homografts.

However, there have been encouraging data regarding use of nonvalved conduits in selected patients with normal pulmonary artery pressure, regardless of the obvious disadvantage of pulmonary artery-right ventricular insufficiency.[15] No long-term data are yet available.

Conduit Replacement

Regardless of the type of conduit originally utilized, the possibility of conduit failure must be considered in every patient. The physicians responsible for making the decision whether to replace a conduit must take into consideration the degree of right ventricular dysfunction induced by conduit obstruction (and/or insufficiency), the risk of the reoperation to replace the conduit, and the potential longevity of the replacement prosthesis. Clearly, the lower the risk of operation and the better the replacement valve, the more aggressive one would be in advocating replacement. Thus, any criteria brought forward at this time would be expected to change as technology improves.

The decision-making process regarding reoperation for conduit replacement must take place in the context of careful monitoring of the patient's status vis à vis right ventricular function, both on a clinical and laboratory basis. A right ventricle that has had an outflow reconstruction was already hypertrophied and fibrotic at the time of the original surgical procedure because of high afterload requirements since birth. Such a ventricle can function at systemic pressure for many years, even decades. However, once right ventricular function begins to deteriorate in the face of chronic obstruction, there may be rapid progression of right ventricular failure, leading to irreversible muscle dysfunction. This can be accelerated further by increasing obstruction, creating still more afterload requirement for the already compromised ventricle. Thus, careful follow-up and reevaluation is an important aspect of management in any patient with a right ventricular-to-pulmonary artery conduit regardless of type or number of years following the original procedure. Reassessment of the patient's cardiovascular status should be carried out at no less than six-month intervals.

An evaluation approach that is useful in assessing the patient's status at increasing levels of more detailed investigation is shown in

---

Table I
Evaluation of Patients For RV–PA Conduit Replacement

History and physical examination	–symptoms –more active RV impulse –increased intensity and length of systolic murmur
Noninvasive studies: (X-ray, ECG, 2D echo, Doppler, radionuclide, exercise)	–progressive cardiac enlargement –increased RV-PA gradient estimated –decreased RV function
Cardiac catheterization and angiography	–all levels of obstruction demonstrated –gradients measured –pulmonary vascular resistance assessed

---

Table I. A change in status as determined by history, physical examination, electrocardiogram, x-ray, two-dimensional echocardiogram, and/or Doppler study requires further assessment. The latter might include exercise study, radionuclide investigation, and then, if necessary, cardiac catheterization.

A final decision regarding surgical reintervention for conduit replacement, as with all decision making, rests on clinical judgment. At the extremes of the spectrum there is no particular problem. A patient with suprasystemic right ventricular pressure and with signs and symptoms, as well as laboratory studies, indicating severe right ventricular obstruction, requires conduit replacement. An asymptomatic patient with little or no obstruction and good right ventricular function can be followed routinely. However, in the "gray areas" of subtle right ventricular performance abnormalities and moderate gradients, the decision as to whether to reintervene may be a difficult one. An approach to this problem based on measured or "confidently" estimated right ventricular pressure indicated by clinical examination and nondirect measurement techniques is shown in Figure 1. It is suggested that patients with suprasystemic right ventricular pressure undergo conduit replacement regardless of clinical status. In this situation obstruction is severe, but right ventricular performance is relatively well preserved, as reflected by ventricular muscle that continues to generate high pressure. Replacement of the obstructed conduit is beneficial and should be carried out promptly before deterioration in right ventricular performance. Patients with

RV PRESSURE	REINTERVENTION*†
Suprasystemic	No other criteria required
Systemic range	Symptoms
	Arrhythmia
	Signs of decreasing RV function
	↑ REVD
	↓ EF
	Associated tricuspid valve disease
Less than systemic; but significant obstruction present	RV failure
	Poor RV function
	Low cardiac output
	Arrhythmia
	Associated tricuspid valve disease
Normal range; no obstruction	†

Figure 1. *Criteria for RV–PA conduit replacement.*
*Consider added effects of peripheral pulmonary stenosis and/or pulmonary vascular obstructive disease. †Bacterial endocarditis may be an indication regardless of right ventricular pressure.

right ventricular pressure in the systemic range should have conduit replacement if there are even mild signs of compromised right ventricular function on a clinical and/or laboratory basis. Arrhythmias must be carefully evaluated in this context. If systemic right ventricular pressure has resulted from rapid progression of obstruction rather than from stenosis that has been stable for a considerable length of time, reintervention may be advisable even if there are no symptoms or worsening of right ventricular function.

When right ventricular pressure is below systemic and function is good to excellent, the degree of obstruction is mild and the patient can be watched carefully for progression. On the other hand, in the face of right ventricular failure and low cardiac output, a lower gradient will be measured even in the presence of severe obstruction. This combination of findings is especially likely to be seen in the presence of tricuspid valve insufficiency. Under these conditions, urgent relief of obstruction is mandatory. Right ventricular performance may be expected to improve after conduit replacement, but in extreme cases, right ventricular dysfunction may be so severe that the patient's clinical course continues to deteriorate, and the prognosis becomes poor. This possibility underscores the importance of frequent and careful reassessment of clinical status in these patients.

The decision-making process becomes more complex in the presence of peripheral pulmonary stenosis or pulmonary vascular obstructive disease when some of the right ventricular work requirements are secondary to one of these additional factors. However, if significant obstruction is present across the conduit, replacement is advisable in order to partially alleviate right ventricular afterload.

As to the selection of a conduit for replacement, the same considerations apply as for the initial operation. At this time, the best reported results are those in which fresh aortic homografts, nonvalved Dacron tubes, or pericardial conduits have been used.[4,15]

Conclusions

Right ventricular-to-pulmonary artery conduits have a variable functional longevity depending on conduit size, type of prosthesis, and surgical technique. Active investigation is being carried out aimed at prolonging the effectiveness of these conduits. However, at present it is to be expected that the great majority will become obstructed during childhood or early adult life. Factors that must be considered in the decision-making process as to replacement include (1) the risk of reoperation, (2) the durability of the replacement conduit, (3) the severity of right ventricular outflow obstruction, and (4) the effects of chronic obstruction on right ventricular function. Criteria are presented based on assessment of the patient's clinical course, right ventricular pressure, and right ventricular function data. Frequent reassessment of patients who are not yet considered to be candidates for replacement is mandatory, since progression of conduit obstruction and dysfunction may occur rapidly.

References

1. Ross DN, Somerville J: Correction of pulmonary atresia with a homograft aortic valve. *Lancet* 2:1446–1447, 1966.
2. Moodie DS, Mair DD, Fulton RE, et al: Aortic homograft obstruction. *J Thorac Cardiovasc Surg* 72:553–561, 1976.
3. Al-Janabi N, Gonzales-Lavin L, Neirotti R, et al: Viability of fresh aortic valve homografts: a quantitative assessment. *Thorax* 27:83–86, 1972.
4. Shabbo FB, Wain WH, Ross DN: Right ventricular outflow reconstruction with aortic homograft conduit: analysis of long-term results. *Thorac Cardiovasc Surg* 29:21–25, 1981.

5. di Carlo D, de Leval MR, Stark J: "Fresh," antibiotic sterilized aortic homografts in extracardiac valved conduits. Long-term results. *Thorac Cardiovasc Surg* 32:10–14, 1984.

6. Somerville J, Ross D: Fate of the aortic homograft used for reconstruction of the right ventricular outflow tract (RVOT) in pulmonary atresia and Fallot variants. *Proc Annu Meet Eur Pediatr Soc*, Bordeaux, France, May 3–6, 1983.

7. Bowman FO Jr, Hancock WD, Malm JR: A valve-containing Dacron prosthesis. *Arch Surg* 107:724–728, 1973.

8. Carpentier A, Deloche A, Relland J., et al: Six year follow-up of glutaraldehyde-preserved heterografts. *J Thorac Cardiovasc Surg* 68:771, 1974.

9. Ciaravella JM, McGoon DC, Danielson GK, et al: Experience with the extracardiac conduit. *J Thorac Cardiovasc Surg* 78:920–930, 1979.

10. Agarwal KC, Edwards WD, Feldt RH, et al: Clinicopathological correlates of obstructed right-sided porcine-valved extracardiac conduits. *J Thorac Cardiovasc Surg* 81:591–5601, 1981.

11. Vergesslich KA, Gersony WM, Steeg CN, et al: Postoperative assessment of porcine-valved right ventricular-pulmonary artery conduits. *Am J Cardiol* 53:202–205, 1984.

12. Haverich A, Walterbusch G, Borst HG: The use of fibrin glue for sealing vascular prostheses of high porosity. *Thorac Cardiovasc Surg* 29:252, 1981.

13. Carpentier A, Nashef A, Carpentier S, et al: Techniques for prevention of calcification of valvular bioprostheses. *Circulation* 70(suppl I):165–168, 1984.

14. Saravalli OA, Somerville J, Jefferson KE: Calcification of aortic homografts used for reconstruction of the right ventricular outflow tract. *J Thorac Cardiovasc Surg* 80:909–920, 1980.

15. Schaff HV, DiDonato RM, Danielson GK, et al: Reoperation for obstructed pulmonary ventricle-pulmonary artery conduits. Early and late results. *J Thorac Cardiovasc Surg* 88:334–343, 1984.

Editorial Comment

Masato Takahashi, M.D.

Truncus arteriosus has joined the ranks of cardiac lesions that are amenable to anatomical correction. Because of the complexity and variability of its anatomy, the truncus continues to offer challenges to the surgeon. This summary addresses the "nitty-gritty" questions regarding surgical management of truncus arteriosus.

Is there an optimal age for truncus repair?   According to the experience of Dr. Kevin Turley of the University of California, San Francisco, the preferred age for primary repair of truncus arteriosus is six weeks. However, chronic congestive heart failure and respirator dependency may force repair to be done earlier. The youngest surviving patient was fourteen days old at operation. Surgery on neonates in the first week of life is hampered by (1) immature myocardium, which is edematous, thereby causing difficulty in suturing in the graft; and (2) mismatch between the smallest available conduit (12 mm) and the available space in the chest cavity. The smallest conduit used by Dr. Turley was a 10 mm homograft.[1]

Although older infants are preferred candidates for truncus repair, infants in congestive failure who are respirator-dependent may not grow and they become progressively poor candidates by delaying surgery due to malnutrition and chronic infection.

According to Dr. Van Praagh's autopsy series, the median age of death for truncus arteriosus was five weeks. It was even lower (10 days) in the presence of interrupted aortic arch.[2,3]

Surgical mortality in truncus related to patient age and pulmonary vascular resistance.   In Dr. Turley's series of patients under six months of age,

233

the survival rate is excellent, but from 6 to 12 months the mortality is 20% to 25%.[1]

There is no question that an elevated pulmonary resistance is a major risk factor. According to Dr. Danielson, among those patients with pulmonary vascular resistance of 8 to 10 units, 85% had pulmonary vascular changes in Heath-Edwards class III and IV. Repair of truncus arteriosus in this group carried a mortality of about 25%. Of the survivors, 25% became worse in terms of pulmonary vascular resistance, 50% remained unchanged and only 25% showed a decrease in pulmonary vascular resistance.[4] Clearly, as Dr. Turley emphasized, the primary focus in the management of truncus arteriosus should be placing a valved conduit as early as technically possible.[1]

When one is confronted with a patient with severe truncal valve insufficiency in association with a high pulmonary vascular resistance, replacement of the truncal valve may be attempted as a palliative procedure without closing the ventricular septal defect.

What is the risk associated with replacement of conduits?   Truncus repair in infancy is palliative and conduit replacement will be necessary. There are individual variations in the longevity of conduits. What is the risk of replacing the conduit? Dr. Turley quoted one death in 84 such operations.[5] Others also have experienced overall low mortality in patients who had only conduit changes. Thus, replacement of an outgrown or stenotic conduit alone appears to carry a low risk.

Can we implant a nonvalved conduit in infancy?   Although nonvalved conduits have been used successfully in other applications, most infants with truncus arteriosus have a very reactive pulmonary vascular bed, which could present problems in the postoperative period. Patients with valved conduits should tolerate a sudden increase in pulmonary vascular resistance more easily. Since all conduits implanted in infancy need replacement with time, placement of small nonvalved conduits appears to have no particular benefit.

How should one manage patients with combined truncus arteriosus and interrupted aortic arch?   In previous years, pulmonary artery banding was done in combination with aortic arch reconstruction. Such an operation carried a high risk. Furthermore, even if the patient survived the first stage, the banding would distort the distal pulmonary artery, making it difficult to anastomose the conduit in the second stage. For these reasons, Dr. Turley prefers a one-stage operation, in which the ventricular septal defect, the truncus, and the interrupted aortic arch are all corrected through the median thoracotomy.[6] This is similar to, though more complex than, the operation for interrupted aortic arch combined with ventricular septal defect.

Surgical management of origin of pulmonary arteries from the descending aorta.   Currently, there are no clear-cut physiological or anatomical criteria for patient selection for operations to correct the origin of pulmonary arteries from the descending aorta. The mortality has been high in a small number of cases at the University of California, San Francisco.[7] Techniques of such repairs are highly individualized. A main pulmonary artery may be fashioned if there exists a confluence of branch pulmonary arteries. If the right and left pulmonary arteries arise relatively close together from the descending aorta, a segment of aorta may be used in reconstruction. However, in most cases the systemic collateral arteries that supply the pulmonary arteries are stenotic. If these arteries are connected to the right ventricle, it would require high pressure to drive the blood flow. This might interfere with postoperative recovery. Thus, full benefit from this operation may be obtained only in the rare patient who has nonstenotic systemic collateral arteries.

References

1. Ebert PA, Turley K, Stanger P, et al: Surgical treatment of truncus arteriosus in the first six months of life. *Ann Surg* 200:451, 1984.
2. Van Praagh R, Van Praagh S: The anatomy of common aorticopulmonary trunk (truncus arteriosus communis) and its embryonic implications. A study of 57 necropsied cases. *Am J Cardiol* 16:406–425, 1965.
3. Calder L, Van Praagh R, Van Praagh S, et al: Truncus arteriosus communis: Clinical, angiocardiographic and pathologic findings in 100 patients. *Am Heart J* 92:23–38, 1976.

4. Personal communication.
5. Turley K, Yee ES, Ebert PA: Total repair of interrupted arch complex in infancy: The anterior approach. *Circulation* 70(suppl I) 1–20, 1984.
6. Personal Communication.

Section V
Controversy in Balloon Angioplasty

To myself I seem to have been only like a boy playing on the seashore, and diverting myself in now and then finding a smoother pebble or a prettier shell than ordinary, whilst the great ocean of truth lay all undiscovered before me.

Sir Isaac Newton

Introduction

Masato Takahashi, M.D.

One of the significant developments in congenital heart disease in the 1980s has been the introduction and widespread acceptance of balloon angioplasty as an alternative to conventional surgery. Benefits of successful angioplasty procedures are obvious in terms of savings in perceived trauma and cost. And yet, as in any newly developing field, there are controversies. These controversies, in particular, surround the subjects of aortic valvuloplasty and so-called native coarctation. Two well-known pioneers with different temperament and approaches present their experiences in this section. These chapters should serve as useful "interim reports" in this new, rapidly changing field.

CHAPTER 19

Balloon Angioplasty for Congenital Stenotic Lesions: Indications and Limitations

James E. Lock, M.D.

The idea that catheters could be used to relieve congenital cardiac narrowing, including valves, is not new.[1,2] There was, nonetheless, little initial interest in the use of angioplasty for congenital heart disease; early angioplasty workers had postulated that angioplasty worked by "squeezing" the soft plaque of atheroma, without actually disrupting the vessel. Obviously, there is no plaque to squeeze in a congenitally narrowed vessel or valve, and thus it was not clear how angioplasty might succeed in children. When postmortem[3] and experimental studies[4,5] indicated that angioplasty might work in coarctation and branch pulmonary arteries, interest in the field quickened. The report that angioplasty successfully dilated a congenitally stenosed pulmonary valve[6] awakened pediatric cardiologists to the multiple possible uses of this procedure in congenital heart disease. This chapter summarizes some of the experimental and clinical information that recently has become available in applying angioplasty to congenital cardiac disease. I will discuss six lesions: coarctation of the aorta, branch pulmonary artery stenosis, pulmonary valvar stenosis, aortic valvar stenosis, pulmonary vein stenosis, and vena cava obstruction.

Coarctation of the Aorta

Experimental[5] and excised specimen[7] studies have indicated the following: angioplasty can dilate a coarctation, although the pressure required for dilation (5-8 atmospheres) is much higher than generally

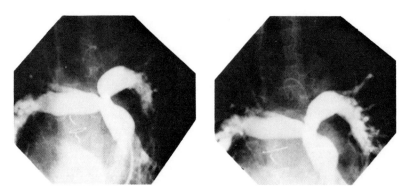

Figure 1. *Proximal left pulmonary artery stenosis, persisting after repair of tetralogy of Fallot, is improved by balloon dilation.*

used for atherosclerotic disease. Angioplasty always succeeds (when it does) by causing a tear in the intima and media, with subsequent healing by fibrosis. With late follow-up, there is no evidence of restenosis. Although no aneurysms were seen in the initial reports, we recently have seen an aneurysm in one sheep dilated over one year previously, suggesting that late aneurysms may be the most pressing clinical concern. Since intimal and medial tearing occur, it is vital not to recross a recently dilated coarctation site with an unguided catheter or wire.

Clinical experience has demonstrated that the native coarctation can be a dilatable lesion in infants,[8,9] although restenosis within a few days to months appears quite common. Coarctation restenosis (Fig. 1) has responded very well to angioplasty,[8,10] without evidence of late recurrence. In general, gradient reductions of 70%–80% have been the rule. Finally, recent clinical evidence[11] has confirmed the in vitro data[7] that native coarctation in older children can be dilatable lesions in the majority of cases, with very good initial results. However, the concern that such lesions might be more likely to develop aneurysms (without a protective layer of adventitial scar) has prompted a number of workers to approach the native coarctation in older children cautiously.

Pulmonary Artery Stenosis/Hypoplasia

Since surgical management of hypoplastic pulmonary arteries has been largely unsuccessful, the advent of angioplasty for this

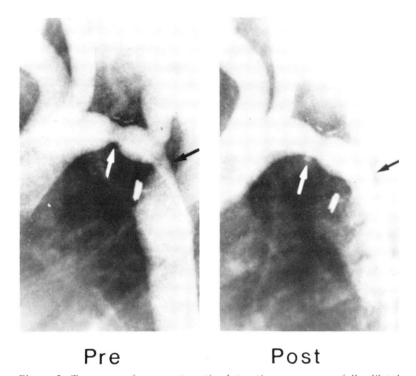

Pre   **Post**

Figure 2. Two areas of recurrent aortic obstruction were successfully dilated percutaneously.

lesion has been particularly important. Experimental studies have shown that the branch pulmonary artery is a very compliant structure, necessitating the use of a large balloon for dilation.[4] Again, dilation succeeds by tearing the intima and media and allowing the pulmonary artery to heal (with fibrosis) in an open position. No late aneurysms were seen, and the dilated vessels grew as the animals grew.

In children, dilation has proved somewhat difficult technically, since the lesions are very distal, and a stiff dilating catheter has to be passed through the heart and past the obstructions. Technical modifications (including the development of a soft dilating catheter, Medi-Tech Inc.) and clinical experience have led to improved results, allowing substantial improvement in the size of and flow through hypoplastic pulmonary arteries (Fig. 2).[12] Significant improvement (as defined by a doubling of the pulmonary artery diameter) has occurred in over half the cases. Late follow-up has demonstrated continued improvement. Preliminary clinical work has suggested that best results are achieved when the hypoplastic pulmonary arteries are long, and when dilation is attempted in children under five years of age.

Pulmonary Valvar Stenosis

Preliminary experimental work has indicated that the pulmonary annulus can be occluded safely for over one minute, and that the hypertrophied right ventricle can tolerate a greater duration of occlusion than can the normal one.[13] In addition, inflation of a dilation balloon in the normal pulmonary annulus does not damage either the pulmonary artery or pulmonary annulus but does cause hemorrhage of varying amounts in the right ventricular free wall.[14] These studies suggest that balloons 30% larger than the annulus (or smaller) cause little cardiac trauma, whereas balloons more than 40% larger than the annulus can produce transmural hemorrhage.

Clinical experience with pulmonary valve angioplasty has been quite good, with over 30 successful cases reported.[6,15,16] There has been no morbidity or mortality, and gradient relief has averaged 60%–70% in cases of classic valvar pulmonary stenosis, although the results in children with dysplastic pulmonary stenosis probably will not be as good. Pulmonary insufficiency has been seen after angioplasty in many of the children, although it has been invariably mild and of no apparent hemodynamic consequence. Late catheterizations have confirmed long-term improvement.

The results with balloon pulmonary valvuloplasty, after only three years of clinical experience, are nearly as good as the published results of surgical valvotomy.[17] If the use of slightly larger balloons produces even better gradient results, and if careful late follow-up reveals no unexpected complications, it is likely that balloon valvuloplasty will replace operative management as the treatment of choice for classic valvar pulmonary stenosis.

Aortic Valvar Stenosis

No experimental or postmortem studies have been reported to date on the extension of angioplasty to congenital aortic stenosis.

Lababidi et al. have reported the results of this technique in a series of children and young adults.[18] The gradient reduction has been good with a very low incidence of aortic insufficiency. Although the optimal methodology for using balloons to dilate that congenitally stenosed aortic valve has not been firmly established, it is possible that dilation of aortic stenosis may also prove a useful procedure.

Pulmonary Vein Stenosis

As there are no experimental forms of this disorder in animals, there have been no animal studies performed to date. Driscoll et al. attempted to dilate such lesions in three children; although the dilations were felt to be successful initially , subsequent follow-up documented the hemodynamic deterioration in each case.[19] The causes for failure in these cases were not clear, and relatively small balloons (6 mm) were used. More recently, larger balloons have been used in these cases, but again the results were unsatisfactory.[20] Although less than a dozen pulmonary vein dilations have been attempted thus far, it would appear that the lesion is undilatable (with current techniques) because it is too rigid.

Vena Cava Obstruction

Initial attempts at dilation of postoperative cava or baffle obstructions were unsuccessful[21] or were associated with early death of the patient.[22] In these reports, relatively small balloons or low dilating pressures were used. More recently, baffle obstructions that occurred after the Mustard or Senning procedure for transposition of the great vessels have been successfully dilated, using large balloons (6–10 times larger than the diameter of the obstructed site) at high (5–8 atm) pressures.[20] Late follow-up in several patients has demonstrated persistence of the gradient relief.

References

1. Rubio V, Limon-Larson R: Treatment of pulmonary valvular stenosis and of tricuspid stenosis using a modified catheter. *Second World Congress on Cardiology. Program abstracts II.* Washington DC, 1954, p 205.

2. Semb BKH, Tjonneland S, Stake G, et al: "Balloon Valvotomy" of congenital pulmonary valve stenosis with tricuspid valve insufficiency. *Cardiovasc Radiol* 2:239–241, 1979.
3. Sos T, Sniderman KW, Rettek-Sos B, et al: Percutaneous transluminal dilatation of coarctation of thoracic aorta postmortem. *Lancet* 2:970–971, 1979.
4. Lock JE, Niemi T, Einzig S, et al: Transvenous angioplasty of experimental branch pulmonary artery stenosis in newborn lambs. *Circulation* 64:886–893, 1981.
5. Lock JE, Niemi T, Burke BA, et al: Transcutaneous angioplasty of experimental aortic coarctation. *Circulation* 66:1280–1286, 1982.
6. Kan JS, White RI Jr, Mitchell SE, et al: Percutaneous balloon valvuloplasty: a new method for treating congenital pulmonary-valve stenosis. *N Engl J Med* 307:540–542, 1982.
7. Lock JE, Castaneda-Zuniga WR, Bass JL, et al: Balloon dilatation of excised aortic coarctation. *Radiology* 143:689–691, 1982.
8. Lock JE, Bass JL, Amplatz K, et al: Balloon dilation angioplasty of aortic coarctation in infants and children. *Circulation* 68:109–116, 1983.
9. Finley JP, Beaulieu RG, Nanton MA, et al: Balloon catheter dilatation of coarctation of the aorta in young infants. *Br Heart J* 50:411–415, 1983.
10. Kan JS, White RI Jr, Mitchell SE, et al: Treatment of restenosis of coarctation by percutaneous transluminal angioplasty. *Circulation* 68:1087–1094, 1983.
11. Lababidi Z, Wu J: Percutaneous balloon coarctation angioplasty. (Abstract). *JACC* 3:531, 1984.
12. Lock JE, Castaneda-Zuniga WR, Fuhrman BP, et al: Balloon dilation angioplasty of hypoplastic and stenotic pulmonary arteries. *Circulation* 67:962–967, 1983.
13. Kan JS, Anderson J, White RI Jr: Experimental basis for balloon valvuloplasty of congenital pulmonary valvular stenosis. (Abstract). *Pediatr Res* 16:101A, 1982.
14. Ring JC, Kulik TJ, Burke BA, et al: Morphologic changes induced by dilation of the pulmonary valve annulus with overlarge balloons in normal newborn lambs. *Am J Cardiol* 55:210–214, 1985.
15. Lababidi Z, Wu JR: Percutaneous balloon pulmonary valvuloplasty. *Am J Cardiol* 52:560–562, 1983.
16. Rocchini AP, Kveselis DA, Crowley D, et al: Percutaneous balloon valvuloplasty for treatment of congenital pulmonary valvular stenosis in children. *JACC* 3:1005–1012, 1984.
17. Nugent EW, Freedom RM, Nora JJ, et al: Clinical course in pulmonary stenosis. *Circulation* 56 (suppl 1):38–47, 1977.
18. Lababidi Z, Wu JR, Walls JT: Percutaneous balloon aortic valvuloplasty: results in 23 patients. *Am J Cardiol* 53:194–197, 1984.
19. Driscoll DJ, Hesslein PS, Mullins CE: Congenital stenosis of individual pulmonary veins: clinical spectrum and unsuccessful treatment by transvenous balloon dilation. *Am J Cardiol* 49:1767–1772, 1982.
20. Lock JE, Bass JL, Castaneda-Zuniga W, et al: Dilation angioplasty of

congenital or operative narrowing of venous channels. *Circulation* 70:457–464, 1984.

21. Waldman JD, Waldman J, Jones MC: Failure of balloon dilatation in mid-cavity obstruction of the systemic venous atrium after the Mustard operation. *Pediatr Cardiol* 4:151–154, 1983.
22. Rocchini AP, Cho KJ, Byrum C, et al: Transluminal angioplasty of superior vena cava obstruction in a 15-month-old child. *Chest* 82:506–508, 1982.

CHAPTER 20

Percutaneous Balloon Aortic Valvuloplasty: Results in 37 Patients

Zuhdi Lababidi, M.D.

Transluminal balloon angioplasty is increasingly accepted as a nonsurgical technique for dilating stenotic arteries in the peripheral, renal, and coronary circulations.[1–4] The recent success of transluminal balloon coronary angioplasty in adults has prompted us and others to apply this principle to children with coarctation of the aorta, pulmonary arterial stenosis, valvular pulmonary stenosis, and valvular aortic stenosis (AS).[5–12]

This chapter describes our experience with the first 37 consecutive patients with congenital AS who underwent percutaneous balloon aortic valvuloplasty (BAV).

Methods

In the past two years, 37 consecutive patients who were thought to have moderate or severe AS diagnosed by auscultation, electrocardiography, pulsed Doppler, and 2-dimensional echocardiography, underwent cardiac catheterization, cineangiography, and BAV. The patients were 2–22 years old at the time of BAV. The mean age was 10 years, and there were 28 males and 9 females. All patients had only AS with no associated cardiac defects. The mean resting peak systolic aortic valve pressure gradient (psg) for the entire group was 105 ± 43 mmHg. Two patients had postcommissurotomy restenosis, and 35 patients had native AS. All patients were premedicated with 0.1 ml/kg body weight of lytic solution (each 1 ml containing 25 mg meperidine, 6.25 mg chlorpromazine, and 6.25 mg promethazine) with a maximum of 2 ml given intramuscularly 30 minutes before the procedure. Percutaneous right- and left-sided cardiac catheterizations were performed through the right groin. Cardiac output was measured by the Fick principle using the LaFarge-Miettinen tables of assumed oxygen consumption.[13] Pressure measurements were performed through fluid-filled catheters connected to Gould-Statham P23ID pressure tranducers and Hewlett Packard 8805 C pressure amplifiers. A pullback pressure recording across the aortic valve was performed, followed by left ventricular and aortic root cineangiograms in the left anterior oblique view. The arterial catheter was then replaced by a double-lumen No. 9 Fr balloon catheter (Meditech), which was introduced percutaneously over a flexible-tip 0.035-inch guide wire.

All balloons used were 40 mm long. We attempted insertion of shorter balloons in some patients at the time of pulmonary valvuloplasty, but found them ineffective because the shorter balloon tended to migrate above or below the valve opening when inflated.[11] The maximal inflatable diameters of the balloons were 10–20 mm—at least 1 mm smaller than the diameter of the aortic valve annulus as measured on the cineangiogram monitor.

To avoid air embolization in the event of balloon rupture, we inflated and deflated the balloon several times outside the patient with carbon dioxide, and then with a 50/50 mixture of saline solution and contrast medium until all bubbles were removed. The balloon also was inflated and deflated once in the ascending aorta to make sure that it was not larger than the valve annulus. When the balloon catheter was introduced into the left ventricle over the guide wire, the middle of the balloon was positioned fluoroscopically across the aortic valve. The valve position had been visualized during the aortic root cineangiography and marked on the monitor screen. At this point, the No. 9 Fr balloon arterial catheter and the 7 Fr venous catheter were disconnected from their strain-gauges and connected together using a Y-shaped metal connector with a syringe on the third end (Fig. 1).

The balloon catheter was then inflated to 120 psi for 5–10 seconds, then deflated quickly if the balloon did not rupture. The balloon catheter was then replaced by the previous arterial catheter. Cardiac output and psg were measured again approximately 15 minutes after the BAV when the heart rate and aortic pressure had returned to prevalvuloplasty levels. A second aortic root cineangiogram was performed in the left anterior oblique view. All aortic root cineangiograms were performed with a No. 7 Fr multipurpose

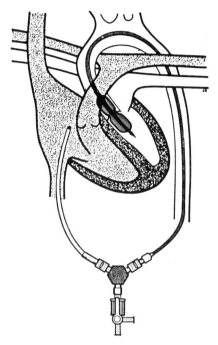

Figure 1. *Heart diagram showing the left ventricular-right atrial shunt when the inflated balloon occludes the aortic valve orifice. The arterial and venous catheters are connected using a Y-shaped metal connector. (Reprinted with permission, Lababidi et al.[12])*

catheter with end and side holes and with the tip about 1 cm above the aortic valve. The arterial and venous catheters were then removed and a pressure bandage applied overnight. All patients were discharged the following morning and return visits were arranged.

Results

All 37 patients had moderate or severe AS with a mean gradient of 105 ± 43 mmHg. With the use of Hunt et al. criteria[14] for assessing aortic regurgitation, mild aortic regurgitation (grade 1–3/5) was demonstrated with aortic root cineangiography in 16 patients. No BAV was cancelled for technical reasons. All patients had an improved psg after BAV. The psg before valvuloplasty for the entire group was 105 ± 43 mmHg, and it decreased to 28 ± 15 mmHg after BAV (p <0.01) with no significant change in cardiac output.

Table I
Percutaneous Balloon Aortic Valvuloplasty
(Unchanged Aortic Regurgitation)
(n = 22)

| | Grade of Angiographic Regurgitation | |
Number of Patients	Pre-BAV	Post-BAV
10	0	0
9	1	1
2	2	2
1	3	3

Table II
Percutaneous Balloon Aortic Valvuloplasty
(Increased Aortic Regurgitation)
(n = 15)

| | Grade of Angiographic Regurgitation | |
Number of Patients	Pre-BAV	Post-BAV
7	0	1
3	0	2
1	0	3
4	1	2

Subjective comparison of the valve opening and jet stream of the aortic root cineangiograms performed before and after BAV demonstrated improvement in the valve opening. Twenty-two patients had no aortic regurgitation or no increase in the angiographic regurgitation after the balloon valvuloplasty (Table I), while 15 patients developed aortic regurgitation immediately after the procedure (Table II). No further development of aortic regurgitation occurred during the past two-year follow-up period.

Pressures of 120 psi were required to achieve full inflation of the balloon. These pressures far exceeded the maximal pressure recommended by the manufacturers of the balloon catheters. At 40–80 psi, the balloon assumed an hourglass shape (waisting) because of the continued resistance of the stenotic valve opening. At 120 psi, the balloon became fully inflated and cylindrical in shape. When the balloon totally occluded the aortic valve, sinus bradycardia and premature ventricular beats developed. When the balloon was deflated, sinus rhythm resumed and the heart rate returned to its level before valvuloplasty within 1–2 minutes. Although the balloon ruptured at a pressure of 120 psi in 23 patients, there was no evidence of embolization or ill effects. Inspection of the ruptured balloons after the procedure showed a clean-cut lengthwise tear in each balloon. On discharge and during the 3–13 month follow-up period, the femoral pulses remained normal and equal with no evidence of arterial or venous compromise to the legs. Although there was significant improvement in the psg in all patients, psg after valvuloplasty was still moderately severe in two patients (65 and 80 mmHg). Both underwent open aortic commissurotomy using extracorporeal circulation, which provided an opportunity to observe the mechanism of balloon valvuloplasty. At operation, both aortic valves were bicuspid with small tears measuring 1–4 mm on the free ends of the aortic commissures.

Seventeen patients have had repeat cardiac catheterization 3–13 months after BAV. In each of the 17 patients there was no significant change in psg or cardiac output between the study immediately after valvuloplasty and the 3–13 month follow-up, indicating persistence of the dilatation. The mean immediate postoperative gradient was 32 ± 18 mmHg, and the follow-up mean gradient was 31 ± 24 mmHg (p <0.01).

Discussion

Congenital AS is a relatively common congenital cardiac defect, comprising 3%–6% of all congenital heart diseases.[15] Although open aortic commissurotomy is well established with a low surgical mortality, it is still regarded as palliative because most patients require reoperation.[16] Percutaneous transluminal balloon angioplasty has been helpful in certain coronary and peripheral vascular diseases and, in our hands, seems to be promising in treating coarctation of the aorta and valvular aortic and pulmonary stenoses.[8–12]

During pulmonary balloon valvuloplasty, the large and stiff balloon catheter may render the tricuspid valve insufficient, thus preventing the right ventricular pressure from rising too high when the balloon totally occludes the pulmonary valve. Because the catheter does not pass through the mitral valve during aortic valvuloplasty, the arterial and venous catheters were connected together outside the body in order to create a left ventricular-right atrial shunt to prevent the left ventricular pressure from increasing too much when the balloon totally occludes the aortic valve. The potential benefits of this are entirely speculative.

Success in increasing the diameter of the aortic valve opening depended a great deal on a high intraballoon pressure and a large balloon diameter almost equal to the valve annular diameter. The shearing effect of the balloon rupture and the 1–2 mm increase in balloon diameter just before the rupture may have contributed to the success in opening the stenotic valve.

High pressure requirement was also demonstrated in vitro on excised coarctation specimens by Lock et al.[17]

To avoid a false change in psg, the pressure measurements after the BAV were performed when the heart rate and cardiac output were approximately equal to values before valvuloplasty. Although the exact effect is not known, and the hypothesis was not supported, using the left ventricular-right atrial catheter shunt outside the groin may have decreased the myocardial or mitral apparatus insult when the aortic valve was totally occluded. The mechanism of relief of the obstruction seems to be a stretching of the valve leaflets and tearing of the aortic commissures.[12] Similar findings were noticed after balloon pulmonary valvuloplasty.[11]

BAV may be an alternative method of treating AS. The advantages are that it is less expensive than open commissurotomy, does not involve sternotomy, and requires only two days of hospitalization. Because it does not involve the use of blood, it may be helpful in treating children whose parents object to the use of blood on religious grounds.

References

1. Dotter CT, Judkins MP: Transluminal treatment of arteriosclerotic obstruction: description of a new technique and a preliminary report of its application. *Circulation* 30:654–670, 1964.
2. Gruntzig AR, Senning A, Siegenthaler WE: Nonoperative dilatation of coronary artery stenosis: percutaneous transluminal coronary angioplasty. *N Engl J Med* 301:61–68, 1979.

3. Tegtmeyer CJ, Dyer R, Teates CD, et al : Percutaneous transluminal dilatation of the renal arteries: techniques and results. *Radiology* 135:589–599, 1980.
4. Spence RK, Freiman DB, Gratenby R, et al: Long-term results of transluminal angioplasty of the iliac and femoral arteries. *Arch Surg* 116:1377–1386, 1981.
5. Singer MI, Rowen M, Dorsey TJ: Transluminal aortic balloon angioplasty for coarctation of the aorta in the newborn. *Am Heart J* 103:131–132, 1982.
6. Kan JS, White RI Jr, Mitchell SE, et al: Percutaneous balloon valvuloplasty: a new method for treating congenital pulmonary-valve stenosis. *N Engl J Med* 307:540–542, 1982.
7. Lock JE, Niemi T, Einzig S, et al: Transvenous angioplasty of experimental branch pulmonary artery stenosis in newborn lambs. *Circulation* 64:686–693, 1981.
8. Lababidi Z: Neonatal transluminal balloon coarctation angioplasty. *Am Heart J* 106:752–753, 1983.
9. Lababidi Z, Madigan N, Wu JR, et al: Balloon coarctation angioplasty in an adult. *Am J Cardiol* 53:350–351, 1984.
10. Lababidi Z, Daskalopoulos DA, Stoeckle H Jr: Transluminal balloon coarctation angioplasty: experience with 27 patients. *Am J Cardiol* 54:1288–1291, 1984.
11. Lababidi Z, Wu JR: Percutaneous balloon pulmonary valvuloplasty. *Am J Cardiol* 52:560–562, 1983.
12. Lababidi Z, Wu JR, Walls JT: Percutaneous balloon aortic valvuloplasty: results in 23 patients. *A J Cardiol* 53:194–197, 1984.
13. LaFarge CG, Miettinen OS: The estimation of oxygen consumption. *Cardiovasc Res* 4:23–30, 1970.
14. Hunt D, Baxley WA, Kennedy JW, et al: Quantitative evaluation of cineaortography in the assessment of aortic regurgitation. *Am J Cardiol* 31:696–700, 1973.
15. Friedman WF, Benson LN: Aortic stenosis. In FH Adams, GC Emmanouilides (eds), *Moss' Heart Disease in Infants, Children and Adolescents*, ed 3. Baltimore, Williams & Wilkins, 1983, p 171–188.
16. Presbitero P, Somerville J, Revel-Chion R, et al: Open aortic valvulotomy for congenital aortic stenosis: late results. *Br Heart J* 47:26–34, 1982.
17. Lock JE, Castaneda-Zuniga WR, Bass JL, et al: Balloon dilatation of excised aortic coarctations. *Radiology* 143, 689–691, 1982.

Editorial Comment

Masato Takahashi, M.D.

To capture in print the status of a rapidly changing field such as balloon dilation angioplasty risks being outdated even before the ink is dry. Nevertheless, arguments as to why a certain lesion is or is not a candidate for balloon angioplasty are worth discussion.

Are criteria for balloon dilation of stenotic lesions different from criteria for surgery? In coarctation of the aorta, the angiographic appearance seems to be more of a determinant than any specific pressure gradient according to Dr. Lababidi. Large collaterals can cause low gradients in severe coarctation of the aorta. It is not easy to quantify what a "dilatable" coarctation is. First, the proximal isthmus segment is not dilatable. Second, the balloon diameter should be significantly larger than the minimum diameter of the coarctation, but less than the descending thoracic aorta. Third, the coarctation should be discrete and the balloon of 3 to 4 cm length to bridge the coarctation, throughout the inflation period.

For valvular aortic and pulmonic stenosis, the same pressure gradient criteria as for surgery has been recommended. Recently, there have been discussions in the angioplasty circles about lowering the gradient criteria for pulmonic stenosis to 30 to 35 mmHg range. In view of the relatively consistent success rate and low risk demonstrated by many centers, this revision of criteria seems justified.

Does balloon dilation angioplasty have a role in the management of tetralogy of Fallot? First, balloon angioplasty appears to be a useful treatment modality in peripheral pulmonary artery stenosis. In addition, a case of bilateral hypoplasia of pulmonary arteries has been treated suc-

257

cessfully with the combined use of surgical transannular patch angioplasty and balloon dilation of peripheral pulmonary arteries. Thus, there does not seem to be any argument about the usefulness of angioplasty in peripheral pulmonary arteries.

Secondly, given the choice between medical management with beta adrenergic blocking agent and balloon angioplasty, some physicians are inclined toward balloon angioplasty of the pulmonic valve if it is stenotic. However, this opinion was not shared by others, including Dr. Richard Van Praagh.[1] The primary problem in severe tetralogy consists of infundibular stenosis brought about by deviation of the crista supraventricularis. In addition, the pulmonary valve annulus is often small, and the valve tissue, although thickened, does not always demonstrate commissural fusion. All of these features tend to make the pulmonic stenosis component of tetralogy a poor candidate for balloon angioplasty.

Can balloon angioplasty be used for discrete subaortic stenosis?   Although a balloon would tear a subvalvular membrane and lower the pressure gradient, the patient would eventually require surgery. Balloon angioplasty may be successful in reducing the pressure gradient but may leave a loose mobile subaortic tissue that would have to be removed surgically. In addition, even after balloon dilation the patient may be left with an eccentric subaortic orifice that could continue to traumatize the aortic valve and may lead to valve replacement.

In view of the frequency of recurrence after relief of discrete subaortic stenosis, even the surgical removal of the subaortic tissue may not offer a permanent solution to the problem, leaving the question of the relative merits of the two procedures less clear-cut.

Utility of the Lababidi Y-connector for left ventricular decompression during aortic valvuloplasty.   Connecting the lumen of the balloon angioplasty catheter to the venous catheter using a Y-connector has received some attention. The limiting factor of such a runoff device is the small lumen of the balloon catheter, which permits only a 0.038-inch guide wire. It is not certain whether such a device has a significant benefit or not. A small potential hemodynamic advantage of such a runoff device may be more than offset by the disadvantage of removing the guide wire and thus destabilizing the balloon during the procedure. Having a guide wire also would permit more than one passage of the balloon across the aortic valve when needed.

Balloon dilation of the stenotic mitral valves.   One group in Japan and a group in Saudi Arabia and a few groups in the United States have performed balloon valvuloplasty in mitral stenosis of rheumatic origin. This application is still new and needs further careful evaluation.

   Balloon dilation of the aortic and mitral valves will probably dominate the attention of those involved in interventional cardiology in the next few years. It remains to be seen whether this procedure will become a standard in selected groups of patients or will be discredited by the practitioners as too risky or unpredictable when compared to the available surgical options.

References

1. Personal communication.

Index to CARDIAC ANOMALIES